Mary Isabella Bryson

John Kenneth Mackenzie

Medical Missionary to China

Mary Isabella Bryson

John Kenneth Mackenzie
Medical Missionary to China

ISBN/EAN: 9783742810557

Manufactured in Europe, USA, Canada, Australia, Japa

Cover: Foto ©Lupo / pixelio.de

Manufactured and distributed by brebook publishing software
(www.brebook.com)

Mary Isabella Bryson

John Kenneth Mackenzie

JOHN KENNETH MACKENZIE,

Medical Missionary to China.

BY

MRS. BRYSON,

London Mission, Tien-tsin;
AUTHOR OF "CHILD LIFE IN CHINESE HOMES," ETC.

WITH PORTRAIT.

SECOND EDITION.

NEW YORK AND CHICAGO.
Fleming H. Revell Company,
PUBLISHERS OF EVANGELICAL LITERATURE.

The Caxton Press

171, 173 Macdougal Street, New York

PREFACE.

IT was on the early morning of Easter Day 1888 that, after thirteen years of active service in China, Dr. Mackenzie was suddenly called to rest from his labours.

During this time he had been used by God in a wonderful way to overcome the great prejudice existing in China against Western medical science, and was the means of founding and conducting the first Government medical school in the Empire.

His labours, indeed, had no small share in giving that impetus towards foreign methods in medicine and surgery which has of late been so noticeable. But while thus singularly successful as a physician, it was in the consecration of all his powers to the attainment of a yet higher end than even the healing of bodily disease that Dr. Mackenzie was specially remarkable.

Few men have kept more constantly before them the spiritual good of those with whom they came in contact. It was ever the evangelistic side of medical work, and the opportunities thus given him to bring to men the healing message of the gospel of Christ, which called forth his enthusiasm, and sustained him amid difficulties and discouragements which otherwise would have been insuperable. When the announcement of Dr. Mackenzie's death was received there was a widespread feeling not only among his own personal friends, but among the friends of Missions generally, that the story of his life and labours would prove helpful to the cause of Medical Missions.

Having had the privilege of the Doctor's friendship from the year 1875 till his death, and been a witness of the wonderful results of his unwearying labours, first in Central China and afterwards on the banks of the Pei-ho, I felt unable to refuse to tell the story of a life devoted, like that of our Divine Master, to the healing of the sick and the preaching of the gospel.

With many other duties to occupy my time and attention, but on the spot where Dr. Mackenzie carried on his benevolent labours, and where his name will for many a year be remembered by Chinamen of every rank with gratitude and esteem, these memorials of him have been written.

As far as possible my aim has been to allow " our beloved physician," by means of his own letters and diaries, to tell of the wonderful way by which the Lord led him.

My special acknowledgments are due to the Doctor's

brother, Alexander Mackenzie, Esq., of Bristol, and to the Directors of the London Missionary Society, for allowing the use of valuable collections of letters. Also to Lieut.-Colonel Duncan and many other friends, both in England and China, for their kindness in contributing letters and reminiscences.

I have throughout received valuable assistance from my husband, who was Dr. Mackenzie's colleague for many years, both in Hankow and Tien-tsin ; and also from Dr. F. C. Roberts, who succeeded the Doctor in the Tien-tsin medical work, and to whom I am indebted for the chapter contained in the Appendix, giving an estimate of Dr. Mackenzie's labours from a professional point of view.

My best thanks are also due to Dr. Maxwell, Secretary of the London Medical Missionary Association, and a valued friend of Dr. Mackenzie's, for his kindness in seeing the book through the press. It is my earnest prayer that this record of a consecrated life may prove a source of encouragement to some who have long toiled for the coming of Christ's kingdom, and that many others may be induced to devote their lives to the bodily and spiritual healing of the millions in heathen lands who have never heard of Christ, the Great Physician.

MARY F. BRYSON.

LONDON MISSION, TIEN-TSIN.

CONTENTS.

CHAPTER I.

EARLY DAYS.

CHAPTER II.

STUDENT LIFE AND VOYAGE TO CHINA.

CHAPTER III.

LIFE IN HANKOW.

CHAPTER IV.

COUNTRY WORK AND PERSECUTION.

CHAPTER V.

LIGHT AFTER DARKNESS.

CHAPTER VI.

PREJUDICE OVERCOME.

CHAPTER VII.

LIGHTS AND SHADOWS OF MEDICAL MISSION WORK.

CHAPTER VIII.

CHANGES—A NORTHERN HOME.

CHAPTER IX.

THE POWER OF PRAYER.

Page

CHAPTER X.

EVANGELISTIC LABOURS.

CHAPTER XIII.

STRANGE PHASES OF CHINESE LIFE.

CHAPTER XIV.

GLIMPSES OF INNER LIFE.

CHAPTER XV.

GROWING IN GRACE.

CHAPTER XVI.

LAST THINGS.

APPENDIX.

CHAPTER I.

EARLY DAYS.

CHAPTER I.

EARLY DAYS.

THERE is not much of beauty or poetry to be found in the English fens of to-day. The great swamps have been drained, and where dark-green alders and golden reed beds once stretched for many a mile around the shining meres we see now a black, unsightly, steaming flat, dotted with scattered windmills for pumping out water, and covered with marshy herbage upon which cattle thrive. The spaces are multiplying where—

> " The land in flowery squares,
>   Beneath a broad and equal blowing wind,
>   Smells of the coming summer ; "

but the process of evolution is not yet complete. The mystery and majesty of the fen-land, of which Kingsley wrote with glowing pen " dipped in colours of the heart," and of which in his early days Tennyson loved to sing, has passed away for ever.

Especially is this the case with that part of the fens through which the Yare meanders with turbid current to the sea, forming by its windings the promontory three miles long upon which the town of Yarmouth is built.

It was in this town that on August 25th, 1850,
a child was born who was destined, in the providence of God, to do so much towards carrying relief
and healing to the homes of one of the most ancient
of nations. Medical Missions, it is true, were no new
thing in China when Dr. Mackenzie commenced work
in that land, but it was those providential circumstances in his career which gave him access to the
homes of some of the highest Chinese officials, which
made his life of such interest to those who watch with
thankful hearts the progress of the gospel in China.
For it can hardly be questioned that the considerable
attention lately given by those filling high positions
in the Empire to Western medicine and surgery had
its origin in the great Viceroy's confidence in Dr.
Mackenzie's medical skill, and is associated with his
work. Before he had reached the meridian of life,
he had accomplished a work the influence of which
on the cause of missions in that land it would be
difficult to estimate.

Could the watchers by the cradle of that little child
have been permitted for a moment to gaze onward
into future years, they would have seen that although
his grave would be made in a foreign land, and he
would "return no more, nor see his native country,"
yet that the environment of his earliest and latest
days would be, in many respects, strikingly similar.
The Chihli plain, on which he would lie down to
sleep his last sleep, and the Norfolk fens of the old
country, have much in common. There is in both

cases the same absence of mound or rising ground, with only a few willows here and there to break the monotony of the scene. The same harvest of reeds in autumn is gathered from the marshy plain, while not unfrequently the high road runs along a bank, to be out of the reach of inundations to which the land is subject. The featureless Chihli plain touches a horizon famous for the grandeur of its sunsets, like the fens of the home land ; and the curious narrow rows for which the town of Yarmouth is distinguished seem to have taken for their prototypes the Chinese streets, along which the name of " Ma Tai-fu " and his wonderful medical skill was destined to become beloved and familiar as a household word.

John Kenneth Mackenzie was the younger son of Alexander and Margaret Mackenzie, his father being a Scotchman from Ross-shire, and his mother a Welsh lady from Breconshire. On both sides his grandparents were pious people, and his paternal great-grandfather was looked up to as an eminently God-fearing man in the district in which he lived. An enormous ivory snuff-box, mounted with silver, with his name and arms and the date of presentation, 1786, engraved on it, is preserved in the family. It was presented to him by the Church members, and is a curious sign of old Scotch habits.

Mr. and Mrs. Mackenzie removed from Yarmouth to Bristol when their younger son was an infant, and it was in that city his boyhood and early youth were spent. Kenneth's father and mother were both

members of the Presbyterian Church in Bristol, his
father being for many years an elder there, till laid
aside by ill health and advancing years. The first
pastor of this Church, the Rev. Matthew Dickie, who
died in 1871, was a powerful preacher and an eminent
Christian. Mr. Mackenzie was deeply attached to him.

In his boyhood the lad Kenneth is spoken of as
being of a reserved, retiring disposition, but quick-
tempered and easily provoked. He was remarkable
in after life for great strength of will and undaunted
courage in the face of difficulties that would have
made many men despair and completely lose heart.

To his Highland blood doubtless he owed a
certain reticence of manner, combined with an inten-
sity of feeling, which in a marked degree characterised
his likes and dislikes. Although not without faults of
temper, he had a very tender and sympathising heart,
and much gentleness and delicacy of manner. He
could be stern at times, but it was conviction and
strength of principle, not harshness of disposition,
that prompted his actions on these occasions.

In his early days he was usually ready to defend
any position he took up with great warmth and
vigour ; for at that time self-confidence and indepen-
dence were not insignificant factors in his character,
and his mind was not of that type which finds
yielding easy.

But as time went on, under the constraining
influence of the love of Christ the graces of the Spirit
blossomed out in his life with such rare beauty as to

form a character of singular attractiveness. Few men, perhaps, have lived a life of such practical holiness, or have been more distinguished for fidelity to their vocation, unworldliness of spirit, and a will chastened by sorrow into glad submission. The ideal of the poet, expressed in the lines :—

"O God, that I could waste my life for others,
   With no ends of my own !
That I could pour myself into my brothers,
   And live for them alone !"

more nearly found its embodiment in Kenneth Mackenzie than in many even of earth's noblest sons.

From his earliest days young Mackenzie was surrounded by holy and happy influences, his home being apparently one of those in which Christian truth is so constantly instilled into the young hearts that in some cases they are unconscious of the moment when the new life in Christ Jesus is born into their spirits, and can hardly remember the time when spiritual things were not a very living reality to them. This was not the case, however, with young Mackenzie. He was accustomed to speak with much distinctness, as we shall afterwards see, of the time of his passing from death unto life, and his definite realization of union with Christ.

His education was carried on, at a private school in Bristol, by Dr. John Stone of King Square ; but he showed little liking for study. There was little to distinguish his early days from those of other boys full of spirits, fonder of healthy exercise than of school work.   He left school at the age of fifteen, and entered business as a clerk in a merchant's office.

During this time he seems to have occupied his spare hours with general reading of an instructive and helpful character, with a view to mental development. He joined some of his young acquaintances in attending various meetings which were held regularly at the rooms of the Young Men's Christian Association in Bristol.

There was a prayer-meeting on Friday evenings, and a Bible-class on Sunday afternoons, conducted by Mr. Thomas Ostler, who writes in affectionate terms his remembrances of the days when as a lad Dr. Mackenzie came under his influence.   Ministers and evangelists visiting Bristol seem to have been frequently invited to speak to the members of these young men's classes, and though without doubt the work of preparation and the sowing of the good seed had been going on for many years before, it was on two of these occasions that Kenneth's young heart seems to have been brought face to face with the absolute necessity of making a definite stand on the Lord's side and confessing Christ before his companions.

He was a quiet, thoughtful lad at this time, of serious disposition ; but he had evidently begun to feel that sense of insufficiency and helplessness at the thought of facing alone the mysteries and problems of human life which comes so often to young spirits on the threshold of life. This painful sense of need proves, not unfrequently, a Divine clue, by the following of which the youthful heart is led into the very presence of its rightful Lord and Saviour, and finds in Him full satisfaction for all its high aspirations.

The first of the occasions mentioned above, which seems to have formed an important link in the chain of events which were blessed by the Spirit to the awakening of young Mackenzie and bringing him to the step of entire consecration to the Master's service, was a certain May Sunday in the year 1867. The subject for conversation at the Bible-class, we are told, was "A Good Conscience," and many of the young men in attendance were much impressed. Before they separated, an address was given by Mr. D. L. Moody, who was then on his first visit to England, previous to the time when he made his great evangelistic tour.

The young men who desired prayer to be offered on their behalf were requested to rise from their seats, and Mackenzie with many others did so. Fifteen members of the class decided for Christ ; but although he of whom we write always dated his earnest desire for a spiritual life from that occasion,—and he was undoubtedly deeply impressed by the afternoon's ser-vices,—yet, as he himself remarks in a letter of a year later, " It was only momentary, and I soon fell away."

It does not seem to have been a very happy year that immediately followed this Sunday when the young man's heart was first awakened to its own helplessness and deep need of a Saviour.

For a considerable time he attended the Association meetings with great regularity, but for some reason found a difficulty in taking the final step of casting himself in simple trust upon the promises of a living Saviour. The leader of the Bible-class seems to have taken a great interest in the spiritual welfare of his young friends, and listened with much sympathy to the doubts and fears they freely expressed to him at the special meetings which were held on their behalf. But, as one of his companions at that time tells us, they often left these meetings with heavy hearts, talking longingly of those spiritual blessings which as yet they were unable to accept as their own. Yet even at this time, though Mackenzie had not found peace and rest of soul, he knew where alone it was to be found, and would often counsel his young companions to "look up," believing that some day full light would dawn.

Sometimes he grew weary with the struggle, in his longing desire to attain not only to nobleness of life and character, but to the secret of life in Jesus.

He tried for a time to repress these yearnings, which it seemed impossible to satisfy, and for a while gave up all attendance at the meetings which had hitherto attracted him so much. But the Holy Spirit had begun in his heart the blessed work of creating that dissatisfaction with self which can only cease with rest in Christ.

The anniversary of the day on which he had been impressed by Mr. Moody's address drew near, and once again Mackenzie was found in his old place in the Association rooms.

On this occasion Mr. W. Hind Smith, of Exeter Hall, London, then a Y.M.C.A. Secretary in the north of England, was present, and had been asked to address the meeting. The rooms were full to over-flowing, and at the close of his remarks Mr. Smith called upon the young men present openly to accept or refuse Christ as their Master. It was a solemn moment for more than one of his audience when, after a considerable pause, Kenneth Mackenzie and several of his companions rose up and avowed themselves followers of the Lord Jesus. One of the young men who on this occasion confessed his faith in Christ, after the lapse of some years, followed his friend of earlier days to China, and is now engaged in work there in connection with the China Inland Mission. He speaks of the joy with which all their hearts were filled as they left the Association rooms on that memorable afternoon, and of how, as three of them accompanied Mackenzie part of the way home, upon reaching a quiet spot on the hill-top they re-dedicated themselves to be henceforth, in the strength of Jesus, true-hearted followers of their blessed Master.

Thus suddenly and solemnly came the answer to all his weary doubts and questionings. For the answer came, and in the only way in which it ever can come to any yearning human soul,—in the Person of Jesus Christ Himself. Mackenzie always looked back upon this day as marking a very real change in his inner life : he was conscious of a voice speaking peace to his heart, the same voice that centuries before had stilled the storm on the Galilean lake.

How frequently have the philosophers of these later days scoffed at what is termed the methodistical doctrine of sudden conversion ; and yet, if Christianity is a life and not a philosophy, in what other way is it possible for it to come into being than suddenly, as all life ever comes? Growth is no sudden thing, of course, and in the Christian life it only begins beneath these lower skies. It is the boundless shores of eternity that see the harvest time of what is here sometimes only a sickly drooping blade. Sometimes ; but this is not as it should be, when the great Sower of the seed has provided all the essentials for the development even here into the ear and the full corn in the ear. Active service for the Master, in whatever sphere the believer's lot may be cast, is the blessed secret of growth in the Christian life ; and immediately Kenneth Mackenzie commenced seeking for opportunities of inducing others to share the joy which filled his own heart.

Together with some of the friends who had confessed Christ with him, he stationed himself on Sunday nights in a crowded thoroughfare, in order that he might distribute tracts to the passers-by. This work was somewhat of a trial to a youth naturally so reserved and undemonstrative, but it seems to have been the service that first suggested itself, and it was characteristic of him to the last that he never shrank from what he considered duty because it was not exactly agreeable to his feelings. "Afterwards," says one of the little party, "we thanked God together for grace given us to overcome the pride which then needed to be crucified."

In September of this year Mackenzie united himself with the Presbyterian Church in Bristol, of which it has been previously mentioned his father was an elder. The story of the change which had passed over him is thus told in his own words :—

"You ask me whether I hope that I really trust in and love the Lord Jesus Christ. In His great loving-kindness unto me, I can now say that I do. My reason for so thinking is that the Holy Spirit has borne witness to my spirit, telling me that I am an heir of God, a joint-heir with Christ, and an inheritor of the kingdom of heaven, and convincing me that the blood of Jesus Christ cleanseth from *all sin.* On May 10th, 1867, when Mr. Moody addressed the Bible-class, I first thought of religion, but it was momentary, and I soon fell away. On the anniversary of that day in the present year, I first, while at the Bible-class, thought earnestly and seriously of my soul's welfare, and determined with God's help to throw off sin and cling to my Saviour. Since then I have continued, I thank Him, to grow in grace."

Opportunities of service seem to have increased rapidly ; as is usually the case when heart and hands are alike ready to do the Master's will.

It was not possible for a man with the strong

nature of the subject of this memoir to do anything by halves. Having come out on the Lord's side, he could not help but take up active work in the harvest field which is the world. Open-air services, lodging-house visitation, and ragged-school work, all engaged his energies. Mackenzie is-spoken of at this time as a leader among the little band of Christian young men with whom he was acquainted. They were all deeply in earnest in their desire to influence the numbers around them who were in ignorance of the love of Jesus, and they were occasionally asked to speak at religious meetings and to preach in the surrounding villages. Eager to gain greater proficiency in public speaking, with the hope of making themselves meet for the Master's use, they decided to commence a meeting for mutual improvement in this respect. The place chosen for the gathering of the little company was a broken-down cow-shed, about two miles away from the town, and the hour five o'clock in the morning : the conditions being, without doubt, sufficiently hard to test their interest and sincerity. They used to take turns in reading specially-prepared sermons, and young Mackenzie's are spoken of by his companions as being remarkably well written, and a great means of grace to them all. The disused cow-house, with its floor of bare earth upon which they knelt in prayer at the beginning of these meetings, thus became to them a training college for service in far wider fields than they had as yet been called upon to occupy. As the result of this preparation, Mackenzie very soon took part in the special services which for several winters were held in the theatre at Bristol.

The labour and study necessary to enable him to take part in these public meetings occupied much of his time and thoughts. The small note-books which he had in use are filled with anecdotes for the illustration of Bible truths, culled from various sources, in some cases being obtained from books, and in others being incidents of personal experience.

It was in connection with these special theatre services that he met with Colonel Duncan, who afterwards became his close friend, and whose influence was used by God to induce him to consecrate his life to service in the foreign field as a medical missionary.

Even thus early in his Christian life Mackenzie seems to have drunk deeply of the Master's spirit, and to have worked and prayed for the conversion of the most hopeless and degraded of his fellow-men and women. In a little diary belonging to this period of his life, interspersed among notes of gospel addresses and illustrations culled from all quarters, we find some graphic accounts of the people with whom he came in contact, and whom he tried to win as trophies for his beloved Master. One of these persons was a notorious burglar of respectable connections, known as " the king of the thieves." This man's story is related as follows in the young worker's diary :—

" I came to know him one Sunday afternoon while

in Tower Lane with Lenington ; we entered a house and he followed us, and I asked him if he would not come to the meeting. As he refused to do so, we both spoke to him about his soul ; he seemed impressed, and plainly told us what he was, and that he would give it up. We left him, and after a time he came into the meeting. A Sunday or so after, he came to the Mission Service of his own accord, and I invited him to the prayer-meeting, but he did not come. But one Friday evening, as I was returning from business, I saw him in Bridewell Street, and he passed me at some distance. I felt unable to go on my way, and, the Spirit leading me, I pursued him, and again invited him to the prayer-meeting. He promised to come, and, God be praised, he did come. After it was over I went for a long walk with him, and he told me a good deal of his past history. He was nephew of Mrs. ——, and had been a member of a Theological Class at Mr. Haycroft's, Broadmead Chapel. At eighteen he began his work of thieving, and was considered very clever at it. He told me he had been before the magistrate, on suspicion and otherwise, two hundred times, but had so eluded them that he had never received more than two months' imprisonment at a time. He had gained hundreds of pounds, but it had never brought him any good, he said.

"He was one of a gang of seventeen thieves who went to Germany, and all but himself had been captured : he had managed to make his escape to France.

He had not been at his old work for two or three weeks, and had been trying to find employment at his trade of joiner, having, during the past six years, always kept some of his tools by him. He said he had quite determined never to take to his old life again."

Another form of Christian service which at this time occupied much of Mackenzie's thoughts, was what was known as Midnight Mission work. This was evidently undertaken in concert with Christian friends much older and more experienced than himself, and, doubtless, for a man so young it cannot be considered a very suitable sphere of labour ; but the very fact that Mackenzie, with his sensitive, reserved disposition, should have engaged in it is a proof of that zeal for the Master's service which possessed his soul even from the earliest days of his Christian life. That he exhibited much tact and wisdom in this difficult work may be seen from another quotation taken from his diary.

"The other Sunday evening," he writes, "Gittens and Lenington brought a whole gang of men and girls from a public-house to a meeting in Tailor's Court. One, by name ——, was the worst of all ; she refused to come inside to the meeting, and waited for her companions outside the door. I followed her, and commenced talking to her about her soul. At first she seemed hardened, and would not answer me, so I asked her about her home, and if she had ever attended a Sunday-school, and then she replied to my

2

questions. Her parents lived at Newport, she said, but she was not willing to give me their address. She told me she lived at Walter's public-house, Broad Street, and said, if she came to the decision to give up her present life and enter the Home she would see me at the same place next Sunday. Not seeing her again for a fortnight, I went with Gittens to the public-house at which she had told me she lived. We saw her, and, before leaving, gave her a tract. Though unwilling to come to the meetings, she seemed much softened. She was only eighteen years of age."

It was after one of the theatre services which have been before referred to, that, in the course of a walk home late one night with his friend Colonel Duncan, Mackenzie first communicated his hope of some day engaging in the Lord's work in the foreign field. They had been detained, for a long time after the service was over that night, conversing with many anxious and enquiring souls. From the earliest days of his realization of life in Christ, Mackenzie's one idea had been to follow his Master closely. He had not a little of the heroic in his disposition, as is seen by his deliberate choice of work which must have been a trial to a nature which was a singular combination of the enthusiastic and the reserved. In the course of his reading he had come across the memoirs of the Rev. William Burns and Dr. James Henderson, and these books seem to have created in his heart a desire, if it proved to be the Lord's will, to serve Christ in the foreign field.

He spoke to Colonel Duncan of this desire, and received the reply : " You are still very young ; would it not be well to go in for the study of medicine, and in course of time go out to China as a Medical Missionary ? "

His thoughts had naturally been drawn towards that great empire because the workers in whose lives he had become interested had laboured there. Mackenzie replied by enquiring what were the cha- racteristics of a Medical Mission, and was told that if he would call upon his friend next day, he would show him a small volume, entitled, " The Double Cure ; or, What is a Medical Mission ? " This little book seems to have made a lasting impression on the young man's mind, since, only a few months before his death, in the midst of his unwearying labours for the souls as well as the bodies of his patients, he wrote a striking article for the *China Medical Mis- sionary Journal* wit the same title. And certainly in few lives was this happy combination more fully exemplified than in his own.

After reading the book lent to him by Colonel Duncan, Mackenzie resolved, if he could obtain his parents' consent, to give up his business situation and begin the study of medicine, with the view, at the end of his course, of going out to China as a Medical Missionary. When he consulted his parents upon the matter they failed to see things in the same light, and were not willing to give their consent to the proposal.

Another Christian friend at this time was Mr. Gordon, of Pitburg and Parkhill, whose wife was the author of the little book which aroused his interests in Medical Mission work.

Their acquaintance had commenced at the Sunday evening theatre services, in which both were taking a prominent part. Hearing of the obstacle in the way of his young friend taking the path in which it seemed to him God had called him to walk, Mr. Gordon proposed that Colonel Duncan, Mr. Steele, a well-known surgeon in Bristol, and himself should lay the matter before the Lord in prayer, asking that, if it were His will, their young friend's desire should be accomplished and all difficulties removed from his path. Towards the end of his life Dr. Mackenzie wrote : " I do indeed believe in prayer. I am forced to believe in it, and say, from practical experience, I am sure that God does hear and answer our prayers."

On this occasion the answer to prayer was not long delayed. It was almost as in the days of Daniel, " At the beginning of thy supplication the commandment came forth ; " for, on Kenneth's return to his home that night, he found his parents' objections had all melted away, and they were quite willing for him to enter upon the studies which were to prepare him for the service to which he felt himself called.

CHAPTER II.

STUDENT LIFE AND VOYAGE TO CHINA.

CHAPTER II.

STUDENT LIFE AND VOYAGE TO CHINA.

UNFORTUNATELY, there are not many details to hand relating to the medical education of the subject of our memoir. The main facts, however, are as follows. In October 1870 he entered the Bristol Medical School, where he prosecuted his studies with success, and at the expiration of four years obtained his diplomas of M.R.C.S. London and L.R.C.P. Edinburgh.

Subsequently, before leaving for China, he still further equipped himself for his future work by attendance at the Royal Ophthalmic Hospital in London.

It was while in Edinburgh obtaining his physician's diploma that Mackenzie formed the acquaintance of Dr. Lowe, of the Edinburgh Medical Missionary Society. He had already felt himself drawn towards China as a field of labour, having been much interested in the memoirs of Burns and Henderson and their work in that land. Afterwards, an address delivered by the Rev. Griffith John, at Colston Hall, Bristol, had stirred his heart and strengthened his desire to devote his life to service for the Master in the far-off

"Middle Kingdom." By this time Mr. John had returned to his work in China, but another member of the Hankow Mission was at home on furlough, and in frequent conversations with Dr. Lowe had laid before him the great need there was for a medical missionary to take charge of the hospital there. Just at that time, stations in various parts of the mission field were in need of medical men, while all the students in connection with the Edinburgh Medical Mission who expected to graduate within the next eighteen months had already received appointments. It was decided, therefore, to appeal to advanced medical students and young medical men, in the hope that some one might be led to offer himself for this service. A letter to this effect was inserted in the *Edinburgh Medical Missionary Journal,* and arrested Mackenzie's attention. He sought an introduction to the writer, and made himself fully acquainted with all circumstances connected with the Hankow work. Just before leaving the beautiful northern capital he spent a long afternoon with his new friend, afterwards a colleague of his own both in Hankow and in Tien-tsin. Pacing up and down Prince's Street they talked over the needs of the station far away in Central China ; and the young doctor seemed to hear the voice of the Master calling him to offer himself, his talents, and his energies for his Lord's use in that great Chinese city. He returned to Bristol with his mind full of the idea, but determined to wait upon God in prayer for clearer guidance in the matter.

A few days after, in the following letter, he communicated his decision to Dr. Lowe :—

" I write to let you know that, after long consideration and prayer, I have come to the determination, I trust under the Lord's guidance, to offer my services to the London Missionary Society for medical mission work in Hankow.

" I have been able to come to this early decision as the result of several occurrences. My friends at home have not raised the slightest objection to my volunteering. I have had two appointments brought before me this very day by professional friends, and therefore it becomes necessary that I should decide at once upon the course I intend to take. The whole matter seems to be so entirely arranged of the Lord that I dare not hold back. I shall be glad to hear from you in reply to this. Will you lay my offer before the London Mission, or should I apply to the Secretary ?

" Once having come to a decision, I shall be ready to enter upon preparatory arrangements as soon as possible."

Dr. Lowe immediately communicated with the Home Secretary of the London Missionary Society :—

" I rejoice to tell you that we have found a most excellent and devoted young medical missionary for Hankow. While a student he has been a most successful evangelist, the Lord having given him many souls as seals to his ministry. He has just passed his examinations as physician in Edinburgh

with great credit. Professionally, he is very highly
accomplished. He has studied all along with a view
to Medical Missionary work, but did not trouble his
mind looking out for a sphere of labour till he had
passed his examinations.

"On the very day he passed he read the notice
about the vacancy in Hankow, which I inserted in
our last Quarterly Paper, and at once came and had
an interview with me. I am very greatly pleased
with him, and I am sure you will be.

"Mr. Bryson and Mr. Cullen likewise are delighted
with the interviews they have had with him.

"He is a Presbyterian, but a most liberal-minded
man, and one who is ready to co-operate with all who
love the Saviour."

A few days afterwards Dr. Mackenzie wrote to the
Secretary of the London Missionary Society offering
himself for the vacant post in Hankow.

"I had better explain to you," he says, "how I come
to be in this position. In the early part of 1870 I
was led, I trust under the guidance of God, to study
medicine with the object of, at the close of my curri-
culum, devoting my life to Medical Missions. I was
in Edinburgh the first week of this month, attending my final examinations at the Royal College of
Physicians. Having been successful and obtained my
physician's diploma, I called on Mr. Coldstream, W.S.,
who is one of the Directors of the Medical Missionary
Society, to make enquiries about Medical Missions.
He informed me of the need of such a missionary in

Hankow, and introduced me to Dr. Lowe. I also saw Mr. Bryson and Mr. Cullen.

" Having become acquainted with all the circumstances of the case, I returned home to consider and pray over the matter. I have been enabled to come to a decision, and hence my letter."

Having made up his own mind upon the subject, with characteristic impetuosity Dr. Mackenzie was exceedingly anxious to have the matter settled at once with the Society, and seems to have left out of consideration the fact that a Board of Directors cannot move quite as rapidly as single individuals. He was intending to be up in Town in the course of two days, and requested an interview with the Board or the Secretary of the London Mission at an hour which he named. Apparently he was himself conscious that he was expecting matters to be arranged with unusual haste, for he adds a postscript to the effect that he would have given longer notice had that been possible, but Dr. Lowe had taken a week to answer his letter ; an unconscionable time, evidently, to the young man eager to have his future career definitely settled.

To those who knew the beloved subject of this memoir in after years, when, under the chastening hand of a wise and loving Father, the fruits of the Spirit had ripened into maturity, and were clearly visible in his walk and conversation, it seems strange to look back at passages in his life which exhibit him in a not altogether attractive light. And yet a faithful and accurate record of the life of even one of the

best of men must not exclude the mention of those
failings and shortcomings which show they have not
yet attained to the stature of perfect men in Christ
Jesus.

That lowliness of spirit was not at this time a
prominent feature in Mackenzie's character is apparent from the fact that he was far from pleased at
the reception he received from the gentleman then
acting as Home Secretary for the London Missionary
Society. He had evidently expected to be welcomed
with open arms, and accepted almost immediately ;
and it was exceedingly trying to his high-spirited
nature to be informed that it would be necessary for
him to appear before a Board of Directors, when his
application would be duly considered. With considerable feeling he wrote to a friend : " Mr. R——
was to a certain extent kind, but I was treated altogether, I thought, as if I had come up to ask for a
special favour, or a situation, at their hands. Self
very much prompted me to have nothing further to
do with the Society ; but I trust, with the Lord's help,
I shall always be able to keep down self, and therefore
hope to go and wait upon the Board on December
14th, if the Lord will."

The day after the date thus appointed Mackenzie
writes : " I saw the Examining Committee of the
London Missionary Society yesterday, and they
accepted my offer of service for Hankow. I had a
most kind reception from every one."

He goes on to ask the friend to whom he was

writing if he considered, from personal experience of Hankow, it would be unwise for a European to begin life in China in the summer. " Now that the matter is settled," he continues, " I should like to be in Hankow as soon as possible, to begin the process of breaking the back of the language."

A fortnight later he writes to the same correspondent, that it has been decided by the Board that it will be in every way desirable that he should proceed to Hankow in April.

At this time he was taking charge of the practice of a medical friend at Shirehampton, near Bristol, and he writes : " I intend to go up to London as soon as I can conveniently resign this post, and shall remain there until April ; then, if no obstacle prevents my leaving, and I see clearly it is the Lord's will, I shall start for China. I am glad Dr. Mullens has specified a time, as it shows me pretty clearly that April is the Lord's time, and I wish, even in the matter of leaving, to have no will of my own, but that the Lord guide me."

With reference to the question of the wisdom of young missionaries going out to their stations, and remaining unmarried for several years, Mackenzie seems to have had a very decided opinion.

" I am afraid I gave you, while in Edinburgh," he writes, " a wrong impression. I told you I was engaged to be married, and this is so ; but I am not anxious to enter into that condition speedily, unless it would be beneficial to the work. Now, most of the friends of the Society specially advised me to wait a couple of years, until I had done something at the language, before getting married. Mr. John, in his letter which was read to me, strongly urged this, as I could then devote more time to study, etc. I myself should also like to try the climate before taking the responsibility of marrying. So that, all things considered, I am very wishful to go out a bachelor. My future wife, I hope, will be, the Lord willing, sent out under guardianship in some two years time. Though, as a beginner, I should like to wait awhile, I can easily understand that when once engaged in the daily routine of work, the language to some extent mastered, the missionary's life must be rather a lonely one; in that case a wife would be a solace and a help."

According to the arrangement previously spoken of, Dr. Mackenzie left Bristol in January, and shortly after his arrival in London had the pleasure of what he speaks of as "a never-to-be-forgotten meeting" with Mr. Moody, who at that time was commencing his great evangelistic campaign in England. It seems to have greatly cheered the heart of the young soldier, who was just putting on his armour for service in the foreign field, to receive words of counsel and blessing from one who, some years before, had been the instrument in God's hands of leading him to more earnest thought concerning the verities of the unseen and eternal.

Mackenzie assisted in various ways, in his few leisure hours, at the meetings held in the great

Agricultural Hall in the month of March 1875, when Sankey's singing and Moody's earnest words were blessed to many souls.

At this time he paid a flying visit to a friend at Trinity College, Cambridge, and was much impressed and cheered by the little band of earnest Christian spirits he met with among the undergraduates. On Sunday evening he gave an address at a Mission Room, after having attended service in the morning at Trinity College, where he heard Canon Lightfoot preach.

The vessel in which it was arranged that the young missionary should sail for his distant sphere of labour was the SS. *Glenlyon*

He had been down to Bristol to bid farewell to his parents. "I left home at 6.30 on Thursday morning, April 8th, after a trying parting with father and mother," he records in his diary. His elder and only brother accompanied him on his journey back to the great city. The two days before the vessel sailed seem to have been very busy ones ; but he again found time to pay visits to the Agricultural Hall, where Messrs. Moody and Sankey were drawing immense crowds, the great building being packed an hour before the time at which services were advertised to commence. "While we waited the choir sung sweet hymns," he writes. "Mr. Moody's sermon was very powerful, full of reality and life. Mr. Sankey sang 'The Ninety and Nine' with great richness and pathos."

These revival meetings seem to have been among Mackenzie's last memories of the home-land on this occasion, since on the morning of April 10th he bade farewell to his brother, the good ship *Glen-lyon* leaving the docks at about ten o'clock. That night saw the vessel anchored off the Nore, and she passed the white cliffs of Dover shortly after eight on Sunday morning. "This is probably the last of England I shall see for some time," he writes ; " the Lord only knows if I may see it again."

It being the Lord's Day, Mackenzie obtained permission from the captain to hold a service on board. On this first occasion, however, none of the ship's company attended, but the young missionary and one other passenger spent the time in reading and talking together over portions of St. Matthew's Gospel and in prayer. " May the Lord bless this beginning, and keep me consistent in the Christian life. O Lord, make me a burning and a shining light to all on board," is an entry in his journal of that day. Among the books which seem to have engaged his attention was Carlyle's " French Revolution." "I have finished Carlyle," he writes. " What a book ! so striking and eloquent. Carlyle is fascinating ! " Other books which seem to have interested him at this time were a volume of Dr. Reynolds' " Sermons " and Macintosh's " Leviticus," which he speaks of as " most instructive." From his diary we find that Dr. Mackenzie threw himself with much interest into the whole life of that miniature world, the ship's company. He made friends with the sailors, and got himself initiated into all the mysteries of signalling. He played quoits with the captain and passengers, and found it "very good exercise." The second Sunday on board his small audience of one had increased to ten, and he writes of being much helped as he spoke to them upon our Lord's conversation with Nicodemus.

He was always a lover of nature, and writes with delight of the lovely moonlight nights and the glorious sunsets on the sea.

On May 7th the following entry occurs in his diary : " It is five years since I left business to study medicine for Medical Mission work. China was frequently in my thoughts ; now I am on my way thither as a Medical Missionary. Surely the Lord has guided me. May I be wholly devoted to His service." On the next Sunday he writes : " I have had sweet communion with God this evening, and have enjoyed much comfort from the study of the Word to-day. I see there are no two courses ; it must be all for Christ, or else the soul gets dead and cold. Doing everything to His glory, and making His glory our object in every matter, then only is there joy and peace. O Lord, may it be thus with me ! " Then, with reference to the service he had been holding on board, he continues : " How fearfully in-different men seem to be to the wonderful truths of the Gospel, and how powerless are those who are not co-workers with God to influence them in any way ! "

The run on shore at Malta was a refreshing change to the passengers wearied with the monotony of life on board ship.

Mackenzie writes enthusiastically of his first view of that island :—" It was a lovely moonlight night, I never saw such a splendid moon ; such a purely brilliant white, you could read easily by it. The pilot came singing out to us from his boat the usual salutation, ' All well on board?' We steamed into the harbour at once ; and a very pretty sight it was to see the town lit up with gas, and the houses and fortifications showing out plainly in the moonlight. With two other passengers I went ashore at 6.30 a.m. in a small boat, with a beak-like prow. We took one of the boatmen with us to show us the way. We passed through Floriana, a small town with one pretty street, to Valetta, the chief town of the island.

" St. John's Cathedral was also visited, full of memorials of the Knights of St. John of Jerusalem ; outside very dingy, but within most magnificent, everything to catch the eye and the Imagination."

The *Glenlyon* reached Hong Kong on May 25th, and Mr. Edge of the London Mission came on board in search of the young Medical Missionary.

Sholto Douglas was at that time visiting the colony as the guest of the Bishop of Victoria, and was holding evangelistic services there.

By June 3rd the *Glenlyon* had reached Shanghai, and on the 4th the young doctor took passage on the *Tchang*, which started early next morning on her

trip of more than six hundred miles up the great
Yang-tse-kiang.   It could not but be a voyage of
considerable interest to one whose heart for years had
been drawn towards China.   So broad is the great
river that for nearly one hundred miles one seems
to be crossing some great inland sea, out of sight
of land.   Near to Chin Kiang the beautiful Silver
Island is passed, with ancient shrines nestling among
the foliage which clothes its rocky sides.   The bold
peaks of Lu-Shan, the famous range of which Li
T'ai Po, a well-known Chinese poet, wrote in glowing
numbers, also attracts the admiring gaze of the
travellers, and the rock islands known as the Great
and Little Orphan diversify the scene.   The *Tchang*
reached Hankow on the evening of June 8th, and
Dr. Mackenzie received a warm welcome from his
future colleagues, Mr. and Mrs. Griffith John and
Mr. Foster.

CHAPTER III.

LIFE IN HANKOW.

The Heart of the Empire—Pioneering Work in Hankow—
History of Medical Mission—Studying Chinese—Chinese
Street Sights—"We have Doctors and Remedies of Our
Own"—Prejudice Conquered—Yang-tse Floods—Among
the Sailors—Union Among the Missionaries—Fever—Visit
to Kiukiang—The Temple of the Dragon King—Resuming
Work—The Preaching in Glad Tidings Halls—
Wuchang—The Temple of Hades—The Blind See—Aim
in Hospital Work—Showers of Blessing.

CHAPTER III.

LIFE IN HANKOW.

HANKOW, the city to which Dr. Mackenzie had been appointed, is a field of labour large and grand enough for the ambition of any man whose heart is fired with an intense desire to proclaim the glad news of salvation to large numbers of his fellow-men. This great mart, with the adjoining cities of Wuchang and Hanyang, is known in the language of the Flowery Land as the "Heart of the Empire." It is situated in the middle of the central province of Hupeh, at the point where the two great rivers, the Yang-tse and the Han, unite. Hankow is the great commercial city of Central China, and the export tea trade is above the enormous figure of three million pounds sterling a year.

The channel of the two rivers is at this point usually covered by a perfect forest of masts, the number of vessels of all sizes being estimated at from eight to ten thousand. The Yang-tse is here more than a mile in breadth, and deep enough at the summer season to allow of the passage of the largest vessels of war and steamers of all trading companies.

The commencement of mission work in Hankow

dates from the year 1861, when the port was opened for
foreign trade, and the Rev. Griffith John, with his colleague, the Rev. R. Wilson, settled with their families
in two Chinese houses, and commenced the daily
work of tract distribution and preaching, both on the
streets and within the walls of their homes. Towards
the end of 1866 it was decided to commence medical
work in connection with the Mission. An hospital
and dispensary were erected, and the lame, the blind,
and those who were stricken with various diseases
which the medical skill of Chinese doctors could not
heal, came in crowds to the foreign physician.

This hospital was successively under the care of
Drs. Reid and Shearer. As time went on, however,
the accommodation provided was found to be insuffi-
cient, and the situation was by no means healthful.

Anxious that the medical work should be removed
to a more suitable neighbourhood, Dr. Reid, the
physician in attendance upon the Hankow foreign
community, who had given his services gratuitously
to the Society from the beginning, purchased and
presented to the Mission a new site. A subscription
list was circulated among the native and foreign
merchants, which realized about 3,000 taels in three
weeks, and this being supplemented by a gift from
the Directors, the missionaries were able to erect a
large and commodious building in a good locality,
thus placing the medical work in the midst of far
more favourable surroundings than it had hitherto
enjoyed.

The foreign community had from the first generously supported the institution, and were quite willing to defray the yearly working expenses. At this time two young native students were assisting Dr. Reid, and there was a good prospect of many more offering themselves for such service upon the arrival of a medical missionary.

Such was the field of labour to which Dr. Mackenzie had been appointed ; and a grand opening it seemed for one desirous of consecrating his medical skill to the Lord's service.

The young doctor reached Hankow in the middle of June, a very trying time to commence the process of acclimatization. With his usual energy, however, he set to work to get his future residence ready for occupation, being in the meantime the guest of his friend Mr. John. It was arranged that he should share a house with his colleague Mr. Foster, the latter taking the lower story and Dr. Mackenzie the upper ; and a few days found him in possession of his rooms, which he soon furnished in a way that was sufficient for his immediate needs.

His first Sunday morning in Hankow was spent at the Chinese service held at the city chapel, three miles from the settlement, while in the afternoon he boarded two of the steamers which at that season of the year always come up to Hankow for tea. "Went on board the *Cawdor Castle* and *Craigforth*," he writes, " and spoke to the men, inviting them to come to meetings on shore. I gave the address in the evening at the meeting held at Mr. John's house, and was much helped."

It should be said in explanation, that although there is an English church in Hankow, service is only conducted there once a day ; but for many years previous to this date an evening service had been held in Mr. Griffith John's house, which was attended by other missionaries, a few people from the community, and a large number of sailors when the tea-steamers were in port.

Monday morning, the beginning of his first whole week in Hankow, found Dr. Mackenzie already in harness, commencing not only the study of Chinese, but regular attendance at the hospital in conjunction with his friend Dr. Reid. While the morning was occupied in medical work, the doctor's teacher made his appearance at 2 p.m., and the study of Chinese commenced.

" I had my first lesson in Chinese this afternoon," he writes. " My teacher, Yang by name, is a very happy, light-hearted fellow, a Christian. I like him exceedingly. He assists Dr. Reid in the hospital, so that we are brother medicals. ˙ He teaches me thus : we sit down together with the same book, he calls over a word, and I try to imitate him ; my mouth is forced into all sorts of odd shapes, and I struggle on. The idea is first to get the proper sound, the meaning afterwards, and then (probably the most difficult) to learn the characters. We go on for about three hours, until I am tired of repeating sounds after him.

"The hospital is a fine, substantially-built, roomy building, very well ventilated and arranged. On the ground floor at the back is the chapel, seating about two hundred and fifty people ; here there is preaching every morning to patients and to any others who may drop in from the streets. In front of the chapel is the dispensary and consulting-room, where the patients are seen, a vestry for the missionaries, and a room in which the resident assistant lives. On the upper story are two large wards, two small ones, and a good-sized ward for foreigners ; the naval surgeon sends his worst cases here. Outside the general building is a women's ward, and two other small buildings, used as schoolrooms, with the porter's lodge.

"Trees are planted all round the building, so that it has quite a pleasant appearance. The reason we have a foreign ward in connection with the hospital is that the community who subscribed a portion of the money to build it stipulated that this should be the case."

Besides his colleagues of the London Mission, Dr. Mackenzie soon sought the friendship of the members of other missions carrying on work in Hankow and the adjoining cities. At this time three other missions were represented there, the English Wesleyans and American Episcopalians having workers both in Hankow and Wuchang, while the China Inland Mission had just secured premises in Wuchang. Dr. Mackenzie describes, with the observant eye of a new arrival in a strange land, his walk of three miles through the native city on his way to visit Mr. and Mrs. Scarborough of the Wesleyan Mission.

" It is indeed surprising to see a Chinese city," he writes ; " the streets are so narrow that no such thing as a carriage or cart could possibly get through. In some of the medium-sized streets I could almost touch both sides by stretching out my arms, and in the widest of the Hankow streets not more than four or five people could stand abreast. Yet these narrow streets are alive with people all day long ; all heavy goods are carried through on wheelbarrows, or on coolies' shoulders. By the aid of a bamboo pole one coolie will carry a tremendous weight, balancing it on his shoulder with the weights suspended at each end of the pole. They carry buckets of water from the river in this fashion. The richer people are carried in sedan chairs, and every one has to make way for them. You will therefore believe me when I say that locomotion through a Chinese street is a somewhat difficult matter. The shops have no windows, but expose their wares directly to the public gaze. For protection from thieves every shop-owner keeps a dog. The Chinese dogs are mostly the size of a large retriever ; they are extremely ugly and savage, but very cowardly. One cannot go about without a stick, for they always recognise a foreigner, and set up a savage howl ; if you have a stick in your hands, however, they take care to keep at a respectable distance , without this they will attack you. To-day I saw a man professing to extract worms from another man's teeth to cure toothache."

We have seen that for many years past, even before he commenced his medical studies, Dr. Mackenzie's heart had been filled with an earnest longing to preach the gospel to those who had never heard it, and until the end of his life the same zeal for the spiritual welfare of his patients and all with whom he came in contact ever distinguished him.

It was natural, therefore, that he should take a deep interest in the evangelistic work of the Mission, and in the infant Church gathered in the midst of a great heathen city.

"The first Sunday of this month," he writes, "I saw the Communion Service for the first time in a Chinese church. There were present from one hundred and fifty to one hundred and eighty men and women, many of whom had come from miles around. It was a very interesting service, so very simple and yet so solemn. There are between three hundred and four hundred members in the London Mission Church here, though it is impossible to get them all together at any one time."

With regard to his own special work of healing the sick, although large numbers of patients attended at the dispensary, many of them being long-standing chronic cases, and others beyond the reach of medical aid, Dr. Mackenzie found a considerable amount of prejudice and distrust of medicine in quarters where

one would have imagined he would have been least
likely to meet with it.

Writing to his brother he says : " You have probably heard something of the tremendous prejudice
which the Chinese have to everything which is foreign.
A marked instance of this occurred soon after I
arrived. One of the deacons of the native Church,
a very good devoted Christian, was taken ill ; he got
worse, and then Mr. John told him that a new doctor
had come out from England, who would probably
come and see him if sent for. At the same time he
asked me if I would go. Of course I was very willing, but the man would not send for me, and told
Mr. John that they had doctors and remedies of their
own. He is a very intelligent man, an earnest Christian, and one very often meeting with foreigners. For
twenty days he was very ill, getting worse and worse,
during which time he had five Chinese doctors. One
afternoon I had a note from Mr. John, written at this
man's house, asking me to come down, as the people
had consented to my seeing him. Mr. John was very
anxious about him, for the man was a very useful
Christian, and could very badly be spared. I went
down at once, and found the man dying ; they had
only sent for me when they thought all hope was
gone. He was in a burning fever, with a temperature
of 103°, with a very rapid pulse, and dreadfully
emaciated ; for he had only taken rice-water for
twenty days, and consequently his weakness was
extreme. I saw that he could not live long unless

the fever was stopped, as he had no strength ; and believing that malaria was at the bottom of it, I determined to give him a large dose, twenty grains, of quinine straight off.   The only objection was that if it failed they would say that I had hastened his death, so Mr. John told me.   However, I did what was right, and gave him the dose, but I was not allowed to give him food.   In the evening they sent to say he was much worse.   I went down, and found the small room crammed with friends, waiting to see him die, while his own family were pulling him about, thinking to prevent his going off.   The man was delirious from the quinine.   I turned all the people out except his wife and son, and managed, after very great persuasion from Mr. John, to get them to leave him alone. Before we left he had fallen off into a sound sleep.   In the morning, on our way to the house, we met his son coming to tell us that he had slept all night.   We found him dreadfully weak, but without a trace of fever ; still his weakness was very dangerous yet ; his friends were willing now to give him anything I ordered, and so we poured in milk and eggs, beef tea and quinine.   Now he is able to walk about his room and enjoy his rice again.   This case has done me good, for it has given the natives confidence.   Since the man's recovery his wife has been taken ill, and they at once sent for me ; she is now all right again. I have also attended the child of a relative who was very ill.   But the Chinese will only come to us when other help is of no avail."

Dr. Mackenzie had arrived in Hankow at the commencement of the rainy season, when day by day the heat was increasing. It was the time of the annual rising of the river, when the current of the noble stream, always strong, increased exceedingly. This year the river banks were completely obliterated, and boats were plying along the streets for hire, that being the only means of locomotion. The frail mud houses of the poorer classes of the Chinese were carried away by the raging current, and the whole of the foreign settlement was from two to six feet under water.

This rising of the waters commences usually about the month of June, and reaches its maximum height in August, after which it again subsides. Though the rising of the water is an annual occurrence, the river does not invariably overflow its banks, but the year 1875 was distinguished as a flood year.

The churchyard and the approaches to the church in the foreign settlement were completely covered ; men were able to swim over the cricket-ground and to go to the bar of the club in a boat. The curious sight of the tops of trees and the roofs of native huts just visible above the water was to be seen on all sides. At this season malarial fever is always prevalent, and it was not wonderful that Dr. Mackenzie thus early in his Chinese career should be attacked by it.

Languor and headache he frequently experienced, but he kept hard at work with his Chinese studies,

and his interest in the sailors of the tea-steamers
never abated. From frequent short entries in his diary
we find that this work among his fellow-countrymen
was blessed of God, and his heart was gladdened by
seeing many of the men coming out on the Lord's
side. The wife of his senior colleague, Mrs. Griffith
John, had for many years been earnestly engaged in
work among sailors, and she found in Dr. Mackenzie
a fellow-worker after her own heart.

Upon arriving in China it is often a great trial to
the young missionary to feel how complete is the
barrier formed by his ignorance of the language,
between himself and the people to whom he longs
to proclaim the glad news of salvation through a
living Saviour. It is then that opportunities of work
among his own countrymen become indeed a means
of grace to the messenger as well as to many to whom
the message is carried.

This was evidently the case with him of whom we
write. When he saw the power of Christ manifested
in transforming the lives of some of the men who
were the objects of his earnest prayers, he was conscious of a more intense longing than ever before for
likeness to His Divine Master, for victory over sin,
and a more abiding sense of Christ's presence with
and in him.

" We had a delightful meeting on board the steamer
last night," he writes. " The captain invited us to
tea, which we had on deck. It was a very solemn
meeting, full of God's Spirit. The captain spoke at

the close, and said that for many years he had been
a Christian, but had never before felt so much that
he was a sinner. The second and third officers both
appear happy in Christ." In another steamer he
speaks of about fourteen men having found rest in
Jesus. " This is the last tea-ship of the season ; may
it be the most blessed ! "

"I have been thinking and praying about a more
complete trust in Jesus," he continues. "I am weary
with struggling against temptation, and feel very many
failures are caused by *my* trying to do these things
with God." " I am rejoicing in *full* trust in Jesus," he
writes some days later. " I have placed myself and
all my concerns in His hands, looking to Him for
deliverance from temptations. I have been so happy
to-day in simply looking up. May my faith fail not!
I feel so helpless and weak, and yet so safe. The life
of simple trust in Jesus is so delightful, such perfect
safety ! "   .

At about this time the Doctor commenced seeing
patients in the afternoon, since in this way he was
able to devote the whole of the mornings to Chinese
study, and he had already begun to feel that the task
of mastering so difficult a language was no child's
play, but required the whole of one's energies to be
thrown into it.

Missionary critics are often found spending their
time and strength in knocking down " men of straw,"
and one oft-repeated objection to missionary work is
the divided front that workers sent out from various

denominations must present to the bewildered eyes of the Chinaman inclined to become a convert from heathenism. A more correct knowledge of missionary life would soon prove this objection to be only imaginary. Nearly all missionary stations have their monthly prayer-meeting, at which workers of every Society represented in the place meet together to plead for blessing upon their work. And as a matter of fact denominational barriers are almost unknown in China, the missionaries being careful to teach their converts that we are all one in Christ Jesus. Dr. Mackenzie notes with evident pleasure his early experiences of one of these united prayer-meetings. "Had a most delightful meeting of missionaries in Mr. Scarborough's house. The subject of a fuller trust in Christ for missionaries and converts was brought up. The Lord's presence was very manifest. I am sure we all felt it was good to be there. The spirit of union is very sweet. The Wesleyans, the American Episcopals (most of them), Inland Mission, and London Mission all join in perfect love."

"I am thankful to God for deliverance from many of my old besetting sins, which when I fought against them had such power over me," he writes soon after. "I never had so much deliverance from sin as I am experiencing now, because I am taking God at His word more. Yet I want complete deliverance, which I believe Christ can give, for even now do pride and irritability rise up, yet not as they once did."

August is usually the most trying month of the summer season in Hankow, the weather being always close, and the heat oppressive. Patients began to attend at the hospital in larger numbers than ever before. The Chinese spoke of it as being one of the worst summers they had ever known, and natives were dying in large numbers. As is always the case in years of flood, malarial fever was very prevalent.

We have already seen that Dr. Mackenzie had suffered slightly from the effects of malaria at intervals since his arrival in Hankow. Towards the middle of August he had a more severe attack, and though he struggled on with his work for a day or two, still seeing patients at the hospital, he had at last to give up entirely. There was no break in the fever for a fortnight, though he was taking heavy doses of quinine twice a day. It was evident that a change from the malarious atmosphere of Hankow had become an absolute necessity. It was accordingly arranged that Mackenzie should take a trip to Kiukiang, a port about one hundred and fifty miles below Hankow, a few miles distant from the slopes of the fine range of the Lu-Shan. The foreign community of Kiukiang had erected a small bungalow far up among the mountain gorges, as a refuge from the heat of the plains. It consisted of two rooms only, the servants of visitors finding accommodation in the priests' quarters of the adjoining temple of the Dragon King.

It was a delightful change for the invalid from

the flooded Hankow plain, to be carried by coolies,
in a mountain chair, through a lovely wooded country,
past well-cultivated fields and smiling villages, till he
reached the steep path leading up to the gorge in
which the bungalow was situated. " At one part of
the journey," he writes, " I found myself partially
suspended over a precipice as we were turning a
point where the path narrowed very much and was
very rugged. However, I sat very still, trusting in
the surefootedness of the bearers ; but the sensation
of relief was considerable when the path became
broader." The bungalow is situated in the depths
of a deep gorge running between lofty peaks. A
fine stream of water, clear as crystal, with great lichen-
covered boulders cast at intervals into its depths,
breaks up the stream into little cascades and water-
falls, forming a scene as refreshing to the eye as the
air is invigorating and healthful to the body.

After a few days spent in this bracing atmosphere
Dr. Mackenzie felt much stronger, though the fever
still hung about him. He decided to return home,
and left Kiukiang, starting with the dawn to avoid
the great heat of the midday sun.

September had now arrived, and autumn, that most
welcome of all seasons in the Yang-tse valley, was at
hand. The cool refreshing breezes are as welcome
as the breath of spring in more temperate latitudes.
The flowers in the garden borders begin to revive
after the fierce heat of the long summer days, and
life and health come gradually back to many a frame

weakened with the close heat of the almost tropical summer.

Dr. Mackenzie was able to resume his fortnightly letters home ; he had not written for some weeks, for with his usual thoughtfulness he says :—

" I could not write steadily while the fever was upon me, and did not like to frighten them at home. I am decidedly better, and quite free from fever, though my strength has not quite come back. I took charge of the hospital again to-day, and found very few patients. My absence has diminished the number greatly, and practically almost stopped the work. Dr. Reid has been in charge, but his time is so much occupied that he has been unable to give much attention to it."

On the great day of the autumn festival, when all business is suspended, and even the sick put off attendance at the hospital to a more convenient season, Dr. Mackenzie accompanied his colleague Mr. John up to the city chapel, and was much interested in the congregation which quickly assembled when the doors were opened. Daily preaching is carried on in most of the Mission chapels in China. Very frequently a shop in the middle of a crowded street is rented, and fitted up with benches as a " Glad Tidings Hall," where the foreign missionary and his native assistant for many hours every day proclaim the way of salvation through Jesus to those who come into the building. No regular service is held, but as the coolies resting from their burdens, the

countryman with his basket by his side, or the pedlar
with his case of cord and tapes, come in for a while,
the preacher, in colloquial fashion, addresses questions
to individuals, and tries by patient repetition to im-
plant in his hearers' minds some ideas about the love
of God as manifested in His Son Jesus Christ. This
new "doctrine," as they call it, is very novel, and
strangely unlike anything the hearers have ever
listened to before. It is with great difficulty that
they grasp any thoughts relating to the unseen and
eternal. The same persons will frequently come day
after day to the chapel, and in some cases the
missionary's heart is cheered by seeing a genuine
interest in the gospel aroused in hearts before dark
and without knowledge of God.

"Mr. John spoke in the chapel for about two hours,"
writes the Doctor. "It was half-an-hour before he
could get one idea thoroughly home to the people,
showing, it seems to me, how useless are ordinary
sermons to teach these people. Wandering through
the country and simply preaching is pure waste of
time, I think. Men must settle down to patient per-
severing work, and if accompanied by the Spirit of
God, one may expect to see great results from it.

"Mr. John has anxious enquirers at the end of these
patient, hard-working services, which greatly cheer his
heart. To-day there were four. One old man, who
was present for the first time, as most of the hearers
were, was very anxious, and although rather sceptical
upon entering the chapel, was at the close of the

preaching eagerly desirous of obtaining more knowledge of this Jesus who could deliver from sin. His
chief difficulty was that he wanted to do something;
he could not for a long time realize that salvation is
a gift. Afterwards Mr. John prayed with him in the
vestry."

A few days later Dr. Mackenzie took a day's holiday in order to pay a visit to Wuchang, the provincial
capital of Hupeh, and the seat of the Viceroy of
the two provinces known as Hu-kwang. This city
is prettily situated, and possesses some attractive
features; it is surrounded by a wall of about nine
miles in circumference, built in parts upon the slopes
of a hill.

It had only been after a prolonged struggle and
great opposition that the consent of the officials had
been obtained to the commencement of mission-work
in this city. Examinations are regularly held in
Wuchang, which is a great literary centre, and the
officials had argued that it would never do for
students coming up from all parts of the provinces to
find the despised Western teachers of the religion of
Jesus spreading their pernicious doctrines in the capital
itself. Not many years before, a determined attempt
had been made to drive the Roman Catholic priests
from the spot, and by order of the Viceroy two of
their number had been strangled. Their graves,
among the rank grass, on a lonely hill side without
the city wall, are to be seen still. It was not wonderful that Chinese diplomacy had made a determined

attempt to wear out the patience of the persistent foreigner, but Mr. John's zeal and importunity had at last conquered ; the London Mission obtained a footing there in 1865, and since that time three other Societies have sent agents to labour there.

Dr. Mackenzie describes a visit which he made to one of the sights of the place, known as the Temple of Horrors or of Hades.

It is situated without the wall of the city. In the chambers surrounding the central hall a large number of groups are exhibited, representing people being judged after death, and rewarded for their virtues or punished for their misdeeds. The figures are mostly of plaster, but the scenes are depicted with considerable skill, and are hideous in the extreme. Here a man is seen thrown on a hill of knives, there he is sawn asunder, tied to a pillar heated red hot, or pounded in a mortar. After passing through these or similar frightful experiences, before a man is born into the world again he is represented as drinking of the tea of forgetfulness, which is sold by two old women, whose stall is erected close by the gates of Hades.

As the days went on, Dr. Mackenzie's hospital work occupied more and more of his time, the patients who attended at the dispensary rapidly increasing in numbers. " I have been very busy, hardly able to touch Chinese study for the last few days, with so many hospital patients," he writes in November. " I have sought ever since coming here to keep the work quiet, simply to keep it going by seeing those who present themselves, but making it as little known as possible, that I may get the chief part of the day for the language. But I find the hospital is growing popular rather too soon. The family of a farmer, coming from a town called Mien-yang, one hundred miles distant, has just arrived here. The two daughters, fine handsome girls of fourteen and sixteen, were brought here just before my arrival; they had cataract in both eyes from birth, and had never seen. We operated upon them; both cases were successful, and the girls can now see well. They are very intelligent, and became deeply interested in the truth. Before they returned home Mr. John baptized them both. On this second visit they came bringing with them their mother, a woman of about forty years of age, who had also been blind for twenty-six years; there was another middle-aged relative with them who had been unable to see for fifteen years; and a large party of neighbours accompanied them suffering from various ailments. The daughters said, though they thought their mother's eyes were affected in the same way as their own had been, they feared since she had been blind for so many years she was past all hope of cure. They had, however, been teaching her all they had learned of the religion of Jesus, and she had come with them to be further instructed in the truth, as she wished to become a Christian also. I operated to-day upon the four cataract cases, and removed a disorganised eye, which was leading to the destruction of the other, in the case of a lad who accompanied this party ; all the cases look well so far." A fortnight after he writes : " To-day I removed the bandages from the eyes of the woman operated upon for cataract. She could tell me I have whiskers,—a strange thing to the Chinese,—and that I wore glasses. Her companion is getting on well, but will require further operative treatment. Of late I have been besieged with cases of eye disease. This woman, her husband, a man of considerable character, and their youngest child, were baptized upon a profession of their faith on the last Sunday of 1875." Writing to a friend of this case, Dr. Mackenzie mentions the woman's gratitude for the relief experienced, and remarks : " The other day she prayed that the blessing of God, the one true God of whom she had learned, might rest upon me for what I had done for her."

At about this time Dr. Mackenzie mentions the case of a literary man who brought a little girl of about twelve years of age to the hospital in charge of two women. " They had come a journey of twenty miles. The girl had a hare lip, which greatly deformed her otherwise nice-looking face. I operated, and, three days ago, healing being nearly completed, she went away with quite a new lip. The father when thanking me went down on his hands and knees, and knocked his forehead against the floor at my feet, which is their way of expressing very deep homage ; of course I had him instantly lifted up, and bade my teacher

tell him that Christianity taught us to kneel only
to God. This man belonged to the literary class, of
whose pride one hears so much. He takes away with
him a very complete knowledge of the truth, and
there we must leave him with God.

" At first there was a great prejudice against foreign
medicine on the part of the Christians living in
Hankow, but seeing I have successfully attended the
chief deacon of the Hankow Church they all come
to me now. This I am very thankful for, as my great
aim is to make the hospital a means of proclaiming
the gospel, and reaching the hearts of the people
through kindness and whatever benefit medically one
can give them."

It was at about this time that a wonderful wave
of blessing reached the Hankow Church. It touched
first the missionaries of the various Societies labouring
there, and a revival of spiritual life was seen in their
midst.

A meeting for the promotion of holiness among
the missionaries here was held at Mr. John's. " Great
blessing received by all present," is an entry in Dr.
Mackenzie's diary. There was quite a revival also
among the native Christians. " We had a very
delightful meeting at the Chinese morning service
to-day. Wei's son and nephew were both received
into the Church, also two others. A pedlar of the name
of Le spoke, exhorting to more courage in Christ's
cause, since we know that we have the Holy Spirit
with us. We ought to imitate the best Christians in

our midst, and not the poor ones. Koh spoke very
earnestly. He is an assistant in a hong, but manages
to give up an hour or more nearly every day to
preaching. Yang, my hospital assistant, spoke afterwards. He referred to the return of the girls who were
formerly blind, spoke of the coming again from their
home at Mien-yang, bringing with them many others
who were suffering in the same way. He used this as
an illustration of how we, having received the Light
of life, should bring others within its reach.

" He mentioned also the case of the boy who had
come with the same party, with one eye disorganized
and the other failing. I advised and removed the
diseased eye, and Yang showed from this that if we
have a right eye or right hand which is injuring us,
we should, as Christ commanded, cut it off and cast
it from us. The Lord's presence was indeed with
us in the meeting. Oh to be privileged to join in
such a work!"

CHAPTER IV.

COUNTRY WORK AND PERSECUTION.

CHAPTER IV.

COUNTRY WORK AND PERSECUTION.

IT is not unfrequently found in China that work among the villages and in the country districts is far more fruitful in results than is usually the case in cities. The country people are more simple-minded, and though generally ignorant are perhaps for that very reason more accessible and teachable than those whose lives are passed in the thickly-populated towns.

Mr. John, who had long felt a strong desire to reach the people living in the villages surrounding Hankow, was anxious to secure the co-operation of his young medical colleague, and frequent visits began to be paid at this time to hamlets within walking distance of the port.

We find some record of these visits in the Doctor's diary. " On Thursday last Mr. John and I took breakfast at 7 a.m., and, together with our native assistant, Siau, carrying a small bag containing a few medicines and our luncheon, started for some of the villages in the neighbourhood of Hankow. It was a beautiful day, and we had a nice walk, visiting all together four villages. When we enter a place we go

5

to the tea-shop, and sit down.   Mr. John then begins
to talk to the people ; all the inhabitants soon assemble
to see the foreigners, filling the tea-shop and crowding
around the doors.   When he has finished speaking, he
tells them that I am a doctor ; whereupon they rush
off, and soon bring out all the sick people in the place.
Eye disease is terribly prevalent, almost every sixth
person having some variety of ophthalmia.   At one
village we held our gathering and treated our patients
in the open air.   We went into some of the houses,
at the request of the people, to see very bad cases.
We walked about fifteen miles, and then came back
by boat down the Han river."

A few days after this the Doctor, in company with
Mr. John, went to eight small villages on the plain
outside one of the gates.   Though within five miles
of the city, they found no foreigners had as yet
visited them.

On another occasion, news of their coming having
preceded them, the missionaries found a barn had
been prepared for their reception, chairs and tables
having been placed there, and tea and eggs got ready
for their refreshment.   In this place they preached,
and saw many patients.   They also paid a visit to
three more villages on the banks of the Yang-tse,
where they found all the inhabitants were vegetarians.
These Chinese vegetarians belong to the strictest sect
of the Buddhists, and the idea which prompts their
asceticism of diet is the hope of winning the favour of
their deities.

Writing to friends at home of these visits Dr. Mackenzie says :—

"We were everywhere well received, and our medicines eagerly sought after. The greatest difficulty is the terrible indifference of the people to the Gospel ; they trouble their heads very little about any form of worship, most of them simply doing homage to heaven and earth. They seemed to me wanting in sympathy for their sick friends. Yet of course God, by His Spirit, can teach the most indifferent, and we have had much joy in seeing already some signs of interest.

"We always, after our visits, find patients coming to the hospital whom we have met in their homes, and in this way we can follow up the teaching. On Sunday two men were present at the chapel from the village we visited a fortnight ago ; both are anxious to become Christians.

"I am now treating two Chinese ladies, one of whom is the wife of an assistant of the Taoutaidel, or chief magistrate of Hankow. I have plenty of opportunities of studying disease in my hospital. Leprosy one gets interested in out here from never, or rarely, seeing it at home, though I am afraid I shall not benefit posterity by discovering a cure. I get some practice in the use of the knife too. To-day I took away a tumour the size of a large orange, growing from the inner surface of the lower lip of a boy of eight years of age. I have just done a satisfactory operation on the eye, giving a man who had been

suffering years of pain and bad sight, freedom from
suffering and quite new vision. To-day I find he has
got an attack of inflammation of the lungs. I do
hope he will get well of this, as he is very greatly
interested in the Gospel, and a nice fellow."

Writing to his father, after receiving news of his
illness, the Doctor says :—

" Probably very few of us realize even some
approach to the true value of Christ's salvation until
sickness comes upon us, or some other form of
trial. But then, when we are trusting in Jesus, we
realize in some measure what a privilege it is when
we find how great a stay and support He is to us, and
how pain and sorrow can be borne with the arms of
our Saviour around us. And yet how ill we requite
His love, by turning away from Him oftentimes, and
getting cold, and unfaithful, and weak, and miserable
Christians, when, if we but put our entire trust in Him,
we should be bright and strong.

" I find how these things are true of myself ; for my
Christian character at home was very unlovely and
miserable, and **undeserving** the name of Christian,
seeing that a Christian is a follower of Christ, and
should be in some measure like Him. But out here,
where I am thrown much alone, I get to know, I am
thankful to say, more of Christ as a personal Saviour ;
and at this present moment, though far away from
you all whom I love so much, I never knew what it
was to have more joy and real peace than I have at
present. What a joy it is to know that you have

such a stay as Christ always proves to be when we lean on Him, and that all of us, in our anxieties, have the sympathizing Jesus to go to!"

In another letter he gives his first experiences of the great festive time of China—the New Year's holiday, and especially New Year's Day.

"The Chinese New Year has just commenced, so all trade is in consequence suspended. Everything is so quiet in the streets that it resembles a Sunday at home. The beginning of the year is the only holiday, you may say, the Chinaman ever gets, so that he looks forward to it with much eagerness. It is the time for family re-unions, and every one tries to get home if it is possible. Wednesday was New Year's Day, but on Monday most of the shops began to close, and people were making their way home. On Tuesday night nearly every Chinaman sat up to receive the New Year. They let off crackers in great quantities all night long, and feast and enjoy themselves.

"Most of the New Year's calls are made on the second day of the year, though many visit on the first of the month.

"On Wednesday we all went to call on Mr. Shun, our chief native preacher, a scholar who came to Hankow with Mr. John at the beginning of the Mission. We all esteem him very highly, he is such a fine Christian character.

"In going along the streets covered with snow we met a few of the early callers, wearing long robes of silk, with their red visiting cards in their hands.

"Mr. Shun was in bed when we arrived at his house,
having been up very late holding a watch-night meeting for some of the Christians in his own home.
However, we waited until he came down, and sat
round the table, and nibbled our cakes and drank
our tea. Most of the Christians whom I know personally called on me on the second or third day. I
find I am beginning to be able to talk to them a little.
Messrs. John and Bryant have been preaching on the
streets during this holiday season, for many of the
people that are shut up in shops at other times are
about now. I only found out they were thus occupied
on Thursday, when, after working all the morning at
Chinese, I began to miss, after tiffin, the change of
employment which my hospital practice gives me,
for it was shut up for the New Year. I called on
Mr. Bryant, with the object of getting his company
for a walk, and found him just ready to go to the
streets to preach with Mr. John. So I went with
them, and sold many books; but as the people would
ask me questions, I found I had to talk also. On
Friday I went out again, but got separated from the
others; but I managed to get on fairly well, and sold
fifty books containing the Gospels explained. On
Saturday I began to preach more publicly, having
arranged a little address, which had been written for
me previously by my teacher, though I did not think
I should have commenced using it so soon."

It will thus be seen that from Dr. Mackenzie's
first arrival in China his one aim was not merely to

exercise his healing art upon the bodies of his patients, but to bring them to the knowledge of that Saviour who was such a living reality to himself.

It was for this reason he felt it of such great importance that he should use every effort to obtain a thorough working knowledge of the language of the people. To its study he devoted himself most faithfully, and in a very short time made considerable progress in its acquisition. "Being actively engaged in hospital work, of which I am very fond, has kept me from wearying in studying Chinese," he writes to his mother. "In consequence, after six months in the country, I am reading in turn with the Chinese at prayers in the chapel ; this I can only do when they are reading in the Gospels, as I have not commenced the Epistles yet. From the first I was determined to learn Chinese. There is no work so useful as that of the medical missionary, but he must combine the two elements, otherwise medical missions are little more than benevolent institutions, like hospitals at home."

During the Chinese New Year's holidays it had been arranged that Mr. John, with Dr. Mackenzie, should pay a visit to Hiau-kan, a country district about forty miles from Hankow, the residence of about twenty Christians, who had recently been received into the Church.

The principal agent used by God in the conversion of a great number of these people was an earnest Christian man of the name of Wei. He and most of his friends spent a part of their time in cultivating their fields, and occupied the spare hours with cloth-weaving, bringing the product of their looms at stated periods into Hankow for sale.

Writing of this man, Mr. John says :—

" Wei, though not a graduate or even an under-graduate in the Confucian School, is by no means ignorant of the Confucian classics, and will often quote them in a way that indicates, on his part, a more thorough appreciation of their meaning than is evinced by many of the so-called scholars. He is a plain, honest, straightforward-looking man, natur-ally endowed with a considerable amount of sound common sense and force of character. No sooner did he become a Christian than he felt that he must be a living, working Christian. He began at once to teach and exhort others, but the fruits of his efforts did not at once appear. We were constantly reminded, however, of his presence among us as a great power for good, and were cheered by unquestionable proofs of his devotion to Christ. It appeared to be his aim to get hold of all his Hiau-kan acquaintances whenever they visited Hankow, and bring them to me. Often has he filled my study with his friends, and often has my heart been cheered by the Christian intelligence, warmth of feeling, and earnestness of manner which he displays whenever he speaks. He is a thorough believer in the Holy Ghost, and never fails to dwell specially on the importance of prayer for the Divine influence, in order to illumine the mind and change the heart. Pointing to one, he will say,

' This friend has heard the truth repeatedly, and knows it intellectually; but he does not understand it—it has no meaning for him. He has not received the Holy Ghost.' Pointing to another, he will remark, ' This brother, thank God, has received the Holy Ghost at last. I have been at him for a long time, but he could not see it. I could do nothing for him but pray. It is all clear to him now. The Holy Ghost has revealed it to him.' Thirteen of our converts have been brought to Christ by means of his prayerful efforts."

Wei had been very earnest in his entreaties that Mr. John should pay a visit to his district during the holiday season, when all his friends were at home. No foreigner had previously visited the place, and Wei believed that the presence of the missionaries might be the means of arousing general interest in the Gospel among his heathen neighbours, as well as be blessed by God, to the strengthening and building up of believers in their holy faith.

"We had arranged to start for Hiau-kan on Monday," writes the Doctor to his mother, " but at the Sunday morning services were surprised to see Wei and his brother among the worshippers. They had just arrived, and told us that, having held meetings in each other's houses for the worship of God, they had been attacked by some of the other villagers, part of the house in which their service was being held at the time was pulled down and the furniture broken, while Wei himself had been struck. How-

ever, he still wished us to pay our visit, and we saw
no reason to alter our plans.

"So at two o'clock on the afternoon of Monday we
made a start, Mr. John, myself, Siau, our hospital
preacher, Wei and his brother, with another Christian
named Chia. We walked ten miles across the plain
to the north of the city, till at about 6 p.m. we came
to a creek, and hired a boat in which to travel
through the night. This was my first experience of
boat travelling in China, and I got it rather hot for
the first time. It was a small boat, the worst he had
ever slept in, Mr. John said ; but we had no choice,
and it was the best we could get. In the centre of it
was the cabin, if you could honour with that title the
small space, covered over with curved bamboos, into
which we crept, and found just room enough to sit
up in. We covered the floor with our native bedding,
and I had just room to lie down. We were not the
only passengers, for we had to take in ten Chinamen,
who all huddled themselves up into this small space.
We had a short service before going to rest, singing
" I am coming to the cross," which Mr. John has
translated. I did not get very much sleep through
the night, for the Chinese were smoking constantly,
and the atmosphere was very impure.

"About nine o'clock on Tuesday morning we reached
the village, which was at the end of our water journey.
I had crept out of our little cot to get some fresh air,
and, while standing up on the small deck approaching our landing-place, the people caught sight of the

foreigner. They began assembling along the water's edge, forming, by the time our boat came to a standstill, a crowd of several hundred men and boys. They were highly amused and interested to see us attending to our toilet. Although the people were greatly excited, it seemed to be purely from curiosity, for they did not attempt to insult us. Mr. John preached from the boat to the crowd lining the shore, and again on landing. We did not know how to arrange about breakfast ; we had brought bread and cold meat with us, but we needed some place to eat it in, and some tea to drink. The crowd increased so fast that it was impossible for us to accompany our native friends into the tea-shops ; so leaving our companions to get a good meal and follow us, we proceeded, with almost the whole village at our heels. For a long time we had a good escort, but we were hoping to come across a quiet country tea-shop, where we could breakfast in peace. But those hopes soon vanished, for we found we were in the midst of villages wherever we went ; the country was hilly and undulating, and everywhere under cultivation. There are no hedges between the fields, but raised banks, and these banks form the paths, but as they are very narrow you can only walk in single file. It was evident that no Englishman had ever visited that neighbourhood, for as we moved along we found people making towards us from all directions, showing themselves above the hills, and quickly hastening to get a closer view. Some of them appeared amazed, and not to know what to make of us ; yet they were quite quiet, only very curious. At last, in as quiet a place as we could get away from any village, we sat down, and ate our meal without water or tea. Yet before we were half through it we had a good audience. After preaching at a large village through which we passed, we reached, about two o'clock, a fine large lake, where we hired a boat to take us across to the village at which Wei's uncle lives. Here we were received very kindly by nearly all the villagers, and Mr. John preached for a long time. We evidently owed our kind treatment, however, to the influence of our friend, the convert Wei. His uncle, seventy-five years of age, and his aunt were brought out and introduced to us. We were surprised to see how well our friend was connected, his uncle and brother being quite important people in the village, living in good large houses. Mr. John preached for some time to the people, who listened very attentively, and Wei's friends were anxious that we should stay the night with them.

"But the crowd which had assembled to see and hear us was so large that, fearing our host would be much inconvenienced on our account, we thought it better to push on.

"We walked on from this village, with our coolie carrying our bedding, a distance of six li. It was about five o'clock. We were within two or three miles of Wei's home, and very tired, when we found the behaviour of the people begin to change. From being simply curious they began to be rude, rushing along-side of us in the ploughed fields, and shouting in great excitement. The farther we advanced the worse it · grew ; from shouting it came to treading on one's heels, and pushing. We turned and faced the people several times, and Mr. John expostulated with the seniors in a way that usually has the desired effect ; but on this occasion they rather encouraged the boys, and were all evidently bent on mischief. Presently, pelting began ; there were fortunately no stones at hand, but the earth being dry, the ploughed fields were covered with hard clods, and these soon began to fly about our heads. At this stage I took off my spectacles, and pulled my soft felt hat well over my ears, which protected me a good deal. Mr. John was struck on the mouth with a hard lump of clay, which made the blood flow freely, and almost caused him to faint ; and soon after another piece cut his scalp at the back of the head. I guarded my face with my arms, my hat well protected my head, and I received most of the blows about my head and body. We still went on, following Wei, who walked like a prince, calm and fearless, with his head up, just his natural self, and apparently not a bit troubled.

"A little way in front of us, in a hollow, was a creek, which we had to cross by means of a small plank bridge ; as we approached it we saw the opposite bank was lined with people. We stopped for a moment to consider whether we should go on, but the leaders of the attack were evidently determined

that we should proceed, wishing to get rid of us over
the creek, which formed the boundary of their district.
Seeing our hesitation, they began to drag us down to
the water's edge ; and at this time we might have
been killed at any moment, for we were the centre of
a howling, infuriated mob of about one thousand men
and boys bent on mischief, and dragging us about in
every direction. We were several times separated.
I was pushed down once, but Mr. John and the native
Christians kept the crowd off me. The people's conduct was explained by their shouts of 'Go back to
Hankow, and preach your Jesus there ; you shall not
come here.' The standard of Christ had been raised
by Wei and his friends, and the devil had consequently
been hard at work, and hence this hatred. This was
a very trying time, but I felt perfectly calm ; no feeling
of anger entered my mind. Christ was a very precious
companion then. We felt no desire to use force in
opposing them, and we had good sticks with us ; but
had we used them it would have been the signal for
our instant destruction, for the mob was just ready to
take advantage of any such action on our part.

"When they had succeeded in dragging us down to
the water's edge, Mr. John set his feet on the bridge,
but as he did so the crowd on the opposite bank sent
a great shower of missiles upon us, showing that they
were determined that we should not cross. So, our
native friends uniting, we made a rush backwards, and
reaching the top of the bank, made our way across
country, and the people did not follow us very far.

"The Christians behaved nobly all through, one man standing in front of Mr. John, trying to ward off the blows. Two or three from Wei's village had bravely joined us, when it would really have been better for them to keep out of the way. We were very thankful to see that none of the Christians attempted to use force on our behalf. We walked as quickly as we could across country, having by this time, of course, forgotten our weariness ; but darkness was rapidly coming on, and we stopped to consult together as to where we should spend the night. Our bedding had disappeared, but it was decided to send a man back to seek for it, since it had probably got safe to the village, our coolie having gone on ahead. It was quite dark, and we were beginning to think we might have to walk all night, when Siau suddenly remembered that a man lived in this neighbourhood who had been in Hankow, and was at that time deeply interested in Christianity. He had been examined by Mr. John, but had not received baptism, as his case was thought to be not quite satisfactory. Siau determined to go on and seek out the man, while we sat down in the dark, for there was no moon, and prayed to our Father in heaven.

"After a while we heard some footsteps approaching, and calling out, found that it was Siau returning with his friend. Would he take us in for the night? Oh yes, certainly ; he was not in the least afraid. We followed him into the village near at hand, which was a large one ; but our friend was not the master of the house in which he lived ; that personage, however, came out, and gave us a hearty welcome. He also declared he was not afraid to take us in. So we entered, and sat down. The room was a large one, but it was soon crowded with people who had heard of our arrival. This was again an anxious time, for we feared our hosts might repent of their kindness ; but God was still with us, and we left the matter entirely with Him. After a long trial of our patience the crowd dispersed. Our host, meanwhile, had set about preparing supper for us, having already made us some tea.

" We now had time to inquire our new friend's name, and found it was Hu. The village contained five hundred families, and, like Wei's village, was a clan, all having the same surname of Hu. Siau was about to tell him our names in return, when our host interrupted, saying he knew us, that he had been to Hankow, and was a patient in the hospital with a sore throat—I was the doctor there. They then brought in supper ; not content with an ordinary meal, they had prepared quite a feast, with a number of dishes— fowl, pork, bacon, pig's liver, fish, and rice cakes, and a large dish each of something like vermicelli broth. I thoroughly enjoyed my first Chinese meal, for we had not had anything to eat since morning. After supper, while sitting talking, we were delighted and surprised to find our bedding arrive ; our friends had found it, and had brought it on themselves ; they were accompanied by some other Christians, who had come along thus late in the dark to sympathise with us.

We spread our bedding in an outhouse where straw was stowed, and then unitedly knelt down and thanked God for His wonderful love towards us, and prayed that this trial might be the means of the Truth spreading rapidly through these villages.

"We enjoyed a sound night's rest, but got up at dawn, and soon the village was awake, and had turned out to see us. Many of the people wanted medicines. They brought one man to me on his bed, with suppuration of the foot, extremely emaciated. I freely lanced it, and subsequently treated about fifty patients that morning. We had our breakfast hastily, and were anxious of course to recompense our host for the considerable trouble and expense we had put him to, but were surprised to find he would not take money; eventually we left a dollar in the hand of a little child. One of the men of the house also insisted on carrying our baggage for us. I would not have believed there was so much kindness and love in the Chinaman's heart, at any rate where strangers are concerned, had I not seen it. Two or three Christians from neighbouring villages had arrived thus early to show their sympathy with us.

"After we had bidden farewell to our kind host, on the way back Mr. John told me some interesting facts in connection with the conduct of the native Christians on the previous day. Siau, the hospital preacher, during the most critical period, when trying to keep the people off, had said, 'You can kill me if you wish, but don't kill my pastor!' Chia, a strongly

built man, who was formerly a constant fighter, was
struck by one of the most prominent of our opponents.
Upon receiving the blow he said, ' Why do you strike
me ? You see I don't strike you back ; you curse
me, but I don't curse you. I'll tell you what it is,
you can hurt my body if you like, but I know this,
you can never hurt my soul ! ' Wei was very quiet
after the attack made upon us ; he was thinking of his
home and family, and fearing that in their excitement
these men would go to his village and carry on further
evil work there ; for, as he said, ' It is me they hate ! '
Before we had heard that his family was safe, he
made a good remark, as he frequently does. ' Do
you think,' he exclaimed, ' that ten thousand such
actions as these are ever going to knock the cause of
Jesus into nothing ? '

"On our homeward march we reached Pch-ching-
tswei about one o'clock, but found it very awkward to
hire a boat there. The people, knowing that we
must get some means of transport down the river,
asked exorbitant sums.

" Finally, through the help of a respectable man who
had heard Mr. John preach in Hankow, we secured a
small boat and started. It rained heavily on the
way, and when at about five o'clock we landed, it was
still coming down in torrents, and we had thirty li
to walk over a muddy plain. However, we each took
a basin of hot rice, and started. I can truly say I
never had such a walk before in my life. There is a
narrow path of stones laid down for the barrows to

run upon in some parts of the road, and without this
we could not have walked ; but these stones were
covered with thick layers of mud. The fields in some
parts were flooded, though quite dry when we passed
two days before. Where there were not stones we
were staggering along like drunken men, as our boots
could get no hold on the road, covered with mud and
slime.

" All Chinese travellers were safely housed for the
night in the tea-shops which we passed, but we were
anxious to reach home as soon as possible. Thoroughly soaked, we arrived at the nearest city gate
at about eight o'clock, and found it locked. We had
to wait a considerable time, and then succeeded in
persuading the official in charge of the north gate to
send soldiers to open it and admit us."

CHAPTER V.

LIGHT AFTER DARKNESS.

CHAPTER V.

LIGHT AFTER DARKNESS.

ON their return from this memorable journey to the Hiau-kan district, Mr. John and Dr. Mackenzie found themselves faced by the question of the advisability or otherwise of reporting their experiences at the English consulate in Hankow. They had no desire to have any person punished on their account ; the difficulty was that this persecution, having been commenced against the native Christians, would inevitably increase in violence if some decided steps were not taken to check it.

Experience had proved that it would be useless to expect to obtain protection for the persecuted Christians from the Chinese officials ; but now that the missionaries had suffered with them, there was a hope that the mandarins might be induced to issue such orders as would enable the Hiau-kan converts to worship God in peace.

This question of the wisdom of appealing to those in high places to exercise their authority in times of persecution, and to shield with the strong hand of the law those who are enduring hardness on account of their faith, has been much debated in many quarters.

Of course, Chinese Christians cannot be exempt from the old law laid down by the Apostle, that "all who will live godly in Christ Jesus must suffer persecution;" and undoubtedly many trials fall to their lot springing naturally out of their surroundings. Petty daily annoyances try their patience; evil reports and accusations are constantly spread abroad, which can only be successfully met by blameless and Christ-like lives.

Occasionally, however, obvious cases of persecution arise, totally different in character from these trivial vexations incident to the life of a believer in Jesus in a heathen land. It is then that the majority of missionaries maintain it is a duty to support their persecuted converts in an appeal for protection; for these hostile attacks are usually instigated by a desire for the suppression of Christianity, and are not unfrequently sanctioned, if not originated, by the gentry of the land.

The result of such an enforcement of the treaty rights of native Christians is usually the quick suppression of an outbreak which might otherwise grow into something much more serious.

These were the motives which influenced Mr. John and his young colleague in reporting their experiences to the English Consul.

Mr. Alabaster, at that time H.B.M.'s representative in Hankow, at once entered into the matter, but confessed to little hope that a satisfactory settlement would be arrived at if an appeal was made to the native authorities, since in several recent cases of insult and injury done to foreigners which had been brought before him, the Tau-tai had refused to take any notice of his appeal.

Two days after this interview with the Consul, Dr. Mackenzie writes as follows :—

"This morning I received a message from Mr. John, asking me to come over to his house at once. I went, and found the Hiau-kan hien, or head magistrate of the Hiau-kan district, in his library. It appears that the chief magistrates of surrounding districts have to pay their respects to the Viceroy at the beginning of the New Year, so that this mandarin was in Hankow at the very time that the Consul's letter reached the Tau-tai. Contrary to Mr. Alabaster's expectations, but in accordance with our prayers, the Tau-tai seems to have taken up the matter energetically, sending for the hien and bidding him go and settle the matter himself. This gentleman seems to have felt considerable anxiety lest he should get into trouble over the affair, for he not only went to call upon the Consul, but, at his suggestion, came with his retinue to Mr. John's house, which was an act of great condescension.

" This mandarin is a fine specimen of a ruler ; he is about six feet four inches in height, and stout, so that in his long silk robes he looked a giant by the side of Mr. John and myself. He had a great amount of energy, and his voice could be heard all over the house. He was willing to do everything Mr. John suggested. He said he was returning to Hiau-kan in three days, and would send to the scene of the attack and punish the ringleaders, we having given him the names of the actual villages concerned and of three of the ringleaders. He said he would also issue a proclamation all through that part of the district. We were to go up in a week's time, by water, to the city, when he would send an escort to meet us, which would accompany us all the way. He said we might depend upon it we should see no other disturbances in any part of his district, but should be able to go everywhere in perfect safety. Everything seems to be coming out just as we could have desired it. We did not wish any one to be punished, but for the sake of the peace of the district the magistrate said it must be done."

About three weeks after their interview with the chief magistrate of the Hiau-kan district, all the official correspondence between the English Consul and the Tau-tai being concluded, the missionaries were allowed to undertake a second visit to the villages where they had been so unfavourably received.

"We took a boat from Hankow," writes Dr. Mackenzie; "very comfortable in comparison with the one on which we travelled before. Leaving about mid-day, we ran slowly down the Yang-tse, and entered the river leading to Hiau-kan in time to anchor for the night. This river is remarkable for its constant windings and sharp bends ; at one point it converts a large portion of land almost into an island, being only a narrow neck of communication   We took numerous walks

along the banks, which were very enjoyable, as the
weather was brisk and cold. Wherever the population was large we attracted great attention. We
were again surprised at the great number of villages ;
as we advanced on our journey the banks were lined
with village after village, and whenever we looked
inland there was the same sight to be seen. Travelling in the country, even more than in the large
towns, I think, gives one an idea of the immensity
of the population, when you see what an extent of
country is included in one district, or hien, and human
life abounding everywhere. We were surprised, at
one part of our journey, to see a large stretch of
pasture-land,—a rare sight in China,—with a number
of buffaloes grazing. Towards evening, within a few
miles of Hiau-kan city, our boat came to a standstill,
owing to the shallowness of the water ; so we had to
postpone visiting the city till next morning.

" After an early breakfast, on the following day, we
started in a sanpan for the city, where we arrived
about ten o'clock. We at once sent our friend Wan
on to the yamen, with a letter and our cards, while
we awaited his return in the boat. We got a good
amount of staring at, as was to be expected, seeing
we had no place in the small sanpan in which to hide
from view, and the people all seemed to know about
our former attack. After our patience had been
somewhat tried, an officer, accompanied by yamen
runners, arrived, and escorted us to the yamen. The
crowds following us were very great, and could only

just be kept back by the officials. Arrived at the yamen, we had an opportunity of witnessing the amount of license given to the populace. The yamen men tried in vain to keep back the crowd which poured after us into the courts of justice, even to the very door of the inner court to which we were conducted, and then a large number stood and stared at the open door, in the very presence of the mandarin, and listened to all that was said. Mr. John says he had never before been so well received by a Chinese magistrate. We were taken into the inner court, next to the private apartments, and the mandarin came out in his official robes and blue button. We had tea brought us—the best I have ever tasted—in the native fashion, without milk or sugar, and the magistrate remained talking with us for two hours.

"On entering the hall, men who wished to speak to the mandarin went down on one knee. Graduates only are free from this ; yet even they are not allowed to sit down properly in his presence, and all others, however rich they may be, have to kneel. We, of course, bowed and sat down. During the interview this official made inquiries about the Gospel, and said he had imagined that the Protestants and Roman Catholics were all one. He remarked further, that he knew something of the Catholics ; they often defended their converts against the law when they were very bad men."

With reference to this part of the conversation Mr. John himself writes as follows :--

"When we called on the magistrate we were asked what we thought of the proclamation which he had issued in regard to this affair. I replied that my only objection to it was that it contained a reference to the Roman Catholic religion. 'But,' said he, 'are you not one and the same?' This question led to a long conversation on the subject, in which I pointed out the difference, especially in our bearing towards the converts, and the kind of protection we claimed for them.

"'Should one of our converts offend against the laws of his country, or in any way prove himself to be a bad man,' said I, 'he would be cut off from our Church, and you would deal with him as with any other subject. All we ask for him is that he be not molested in the exercise of his religion.' 'If that be so,' said he, 'you must be different from the Roman Catholics! What would you like me to do, and what alterations would you have me make in the proclamation?' He then sent for his secretary, and ordered him to write out new copies and hand them to me. When we arrived at the village where most of our converts live I found that some of them were threatened with dire calamities by their relations if they did not abandon the new faith at once. Seeing that most of this opposition sprang from ignorance, I wrote a letter to the magistrate stating the facts of the case, and requesting him to issue another proclamation embodying such and such sentiments. Early next morning I received four copies of a proclamation, which, to my surprise, I found to be little else than my own letter issued in an official form."

Dr. Mackenzie continues the narrative as follows:—

" The magistrate made inquiries about my work, and showed us every kindness. When we were leaving he charged two yamen runners to accompany us to the Wei village, and himself escorted us to the outer gate of the yamen, wishing us good-bye in the sight of the assembled people. It was a beautiful day, and we were glad to leave the city behind us and enter the open country. With our escort we formed quite a little party. After going some distance we met two other yamen runners, who had been sent to Peh-ching-tswei to protect us if we had come that way ; and we were told the mandarin had also sent messengers in the direction of Tsai-tien, thinking we might come that way. We found the country here, as elsewhere, cultivated on every side, and thickly populated. As we neared the Wei village we noticed the people became much more excited, rushing hither and thither, and crying out ; they seemed to be full of life and energy.

" Several members of the Wei family came out to meet us, and led us into the village. We entered one of the houses, for we were rather tired with the walk in the hot sun ; but we soon found it was impossible to remain indoors, so great was the excitement and curiosity on the part of the people. We therefore quickly went out again, and walked about, giving the people an opportunity of staring at us to their hearts' content. Preaching was quite out of the question, of course, although the people kept calling out to us to ' preach the book ; ' but every time Mr. John attempted to do it, he had to close very quickly, since it was evident the people had not yet satisfied their curiosity, and in consequence could not keep quiet. We were quite a marvel to the villagers, for, with the exception of our own friends, who were in the habit of coming to Hankow, none of them had seen a foreigner before. Whenever we entered the house of a convert a crowd would at once follow, and swarm all over the place. After dark it was just the same, for up to nine o'clock large parties kept coming from distant villages, and persisted in entering the house where we were, to stare at us. We found that the owner of a house in these parts has little control over it. It was very wearying, as we were both tired and hungry, having had nothing to eat since our light breakfast at 7 a.m. until 9 p.m.

" The people were not always content to use merely their eyes ; they wanted to feel our clothes. I found one old woman lifting up the lower edge of my trousers to see what I had underneath. Our boots attracted a great deal of attention, and my spectacles. Not that spectacles were strange to them ; the small size only amazed them, as compared with their goggles. Many of them remarked that Mr. John was a Chinaman, his hair and eyes being quite black, and from his having no whiskers, but black moustache and pointed beard. Moreover, they noticed the case and accuracy with which he speaks Chinese. But there was no doubt in their minds about me ; I was certainly a foreigner—my light hair, whiskers, and eyes were evidently quite opposed to the Chinese idea of things.

" Next day platforms used by travelling actors for stage plays were brought out, and fixed up for our use, and then, with immense crowds in every direction, Mr. John was enabled to preach till he was hoarse. Sleeping at night in the mud huts of the people was anything but agreeable. We got them to place boards on tressels for us, but were kept awake at night by the rats running over our heads. At one meal our host, thinking to give us something done in foreign style which we should like, cooked a lot of eggs, stripped off their shells, cut them up, and put them into a strong syrup made of sugar and hot water. This, you may imagine, was hardly after our taste, but when you are hungry you do not look at what you eat.

" The villagers here are the finest lot of men I have yet seen in China, and Mr. John has never seen finer ; they are athletic, manly, fearless, and simple. Those who have become Christians are very fine fellows, letting everybody know about it when it is almost ruin to them."

With reference to this visit Mr. John also writes :—

" The Christians were delighted to see us among them, and did all they could to make our visit a happy one to ourselves and a blessing to their heathen neighbours. Accompanied by some of them we visited all the surrounding villages, and preached the Gospel to thousands of men and women who had never seen a foreigner before. In several of the villages platforms were raised for us, and immense congregations gathered to see and listen to our message. In one village there must have been two thousand people at least, and the sight reminded me of those grand open-air meetings held amid the mountains of my native Wales, which I have often attended, and which used to have such charms for me in days gone by. The curiosity of the people had been fairly excited, and everywhere crowds of men, women, and children were waiting our arrival. We had splendid opportunities of making the truth widely known, and we availed ourselves of them to the utmost extent of our power. I must have preached a dozen times at least on the second day of our arrival, for we commenced with the rising sun and continued long after the lamp of light had sunk and the cloudy veil of night been drawn. We made it a special point to call at the villages where we had been molested, and preach the gospel of peace and good-will to the inhabitants. At first the villagers appeared shy and guilty, but after full explanation of principles and intentions on our part, and many expressions of regret on theirs, much of this timidity passed away ; and we took our leave of them feeling assured that they knew us better and cherished more kindly feelings towards us."

It is interesting to know that the work, which was begun amid great opposition in this place, where the missionaries' lives had been in imminent danger, has been greatly blessed of God. As so often before in the history of the Church of Christ, so now, the very action taken by its opponents to suppress the religion of Jesus seemed in the end rather to give it a larger entrance. As Dr. Mackenzie himself wrote : " I can only give the result of that visit in a verse of Faber's :—

> ' All that Thou blessest turns to good,
>   And unblest good to ill ;
> And all is right that seems most wrong,
>   If it be Thy sweet will.' "

About two years after this visit Mr. John was able to write : " I have just returned from the district of Hiau-kan, where my heart was greatly cheered. The village is likely to become a Christian village." Some time after, two chapels were built in this district, with funds raised by the country people themselves and the help of other native Christians in Hankow ; the villagers gave also much of their time and labour to the work of raising these little sanctuaries for the worship of the true God. As lately as 1889 we find that the converts to Christianity in this neighbourhood continue to grow in numbers, and every year, through the blessing of the Lord of the harvest, sees the progress to be more marked, new centres of work being added to the old, and houses for the worship of God being erected there.

CHAPTER VI.

PREJUDICE OVERCOME.

CHAPTER VI.

PREJUDICE OVERCOME.

AS time went on, the fame of the skilful Western surgeon spread far and wide throughout the province of Hupeh, and patients came in to Hankow from great distances, seeking relief at the hospital. Many diseases which had hitherto been considered incurable were healed, and the patients returned home rejoicing. Not a few in the last stages of fatal sickness were brought to the dispensary, and when they were informed that nothing could be done for them, their friends still showed great unwillingness to carry them away, pleading with much earnestness that they might not be sent away unhealed.

Rumour does not minimize the wonders performed by foreign medical skill, and cases are not unknown where the physician has been summoned even after death had actually taken place, with the idea, apparently, that one could never tell what was within the power of these strange foreign doctors.

In China medical theories are so closely associated with a knowledge of letters that most literary men are supposed to have some acquaintance with the healing art ; and when official employment fails, many of them turn to medicine as a means of support. Medical knowledge is handed down from father to son in the shape of carefully-gathered prescriptions for the cure of certain well-known diseases. Writing on this subject Dr. Mackenzie says :—

"Chinese doctors profess to be able to diagnose disease by the state of the pulse only. Their knowledge of anatomy and physiology is almost nil ; yet in place of exact knowledge they substitute the most absurd theories. The nature of disease being unknown, they attribute to the influence of the ' five elements ' the onset of disease. To a large extent the physiological action of drugs is unknown, and most wonderful healing properties are attributed to such substances as dragons' teeth, fossils, tiger bones, pearls, etc.

"A Chinese doctor examines the pulse of each wrist of his patient with much solemnity, the sick person's hand resting meantime upon a cushion, while the friends stand round watching the operation with much awe. The tongue is then examined, and a prescription written out; the doctor then departs, after giving his diagnosis and going into long explanations of what is taking place in his patient's interior. Many of the Chinese wonder much that foreign physicians should make so many enquiries of their patients ; they think that they should be able to find out all about such matters from the condition of the pulse.

"Moreover, superstitious notions and practices control and pervert medicine. In almost every case of sickness, idols, astrologers, and fortune-tellers are consulted. Disease is generally attributed to the anger of the gods, or to a visitation of evil spirits ; the priests indeed teach this for their own ends. Charms are in general use to expel evil spirits and pacify the offended gods, and many idolatrous rites are employed. The noise of gongs and fire-crackers used in these observances is constantly heard, and of necessity proves very injurious to a patient whose nervous system is weakened by disease. The charms are written out and pasted about the sick-room ; sometimes these marvellous pieces of paper are burned, and the ashes used to make a decoction, which the patient is ordered to drink. It is not wonderful, therefore, that, medical science being in so unsatisfactory a state in China, the cures wrought by the foreign doctors seem to the people little short of miraculous ; and in many cases the difficulty is not to get the people to believe in the foreign medical man, but rather for them to understand there is a limit to his healing power."

"What faith some of these people have in the knife!" writes Dr. Mackenzie. ."A patient in the hospital with great tumours on his face daily pleads to be operated upon, and the friend who accompanies him seconds his entreaties. Another man has brought in a son who is weak-minded, and begs that he may be healed. They came from a long distance in the country, and the man's disappointment was keen

when he found nothing could be done for his boy.
The father remained in Hankow for some time, however, to learn the doctrine, and became a sincere
believer in the Lord Jesus Christ, and an earnest
worker among his fellow-countrymen."

Another interesting case was that of a Master of
Arts living in the province of Kwei-chow, more than
one thousand miles from Hankow. It was necessary
for this gentleman to visit Peking and appear before
the Emperor, and he was much distressed by the fact
that he had a hare-lip. Hearing of the wonders
wrought by foreign surgical skill, he journeyed to
Hankow, and was greatly delighted by the cure that
was effected upon him.

A curious idea prevalent among the Chinese is that
a spirit can wield much greater power when separated
from the body ; and this is one of the reasons why
ancestral worship is so closely bound up with the
people's life. On this account persons desiring to
take vengeance upon their enemies will frequently
commit suicide in order to obtain their end. This is
a sure means of bringing down punishment upon the
head of the enemy, since the magistrate will hold
him responsible for the death, on the principle that if
it had not been for the quarrel the man would not
have died.

A military mandarin, who had betrayed a trust
confided to him by a friend during his absence from
home, was accused at the yamen of his crime ; the
petitioner immediately left the court of justice and

drowned himself in the Yang-tse, the sequel being that the accused was at once beheaded.

Characteristically Chinese, therefore, was the case of a boatman, who, at this time, appeared at the Hankow hospital with a circular wound, the size of a shilling, opening into his windpipe.

The story he told was as follows. Being in destitute circumstances, his wife sold their little boy, only six years of age, to a stranger, without the knowledge of the father. Upon discovering what his wife had done the man was very angry. He sought out the purchaser, and demanded from him the restoration of his child. The man took no notice of the father's importunities, and expressed his intention of retaining the little boy. As a last resource, the parent determined to try what effect an attempt to cut his own throat would have as a means towards frightening the purchaser of his child into compliance with his request. The stratagem proved to be completely successful, since, fearing that the matter might end in his being required to forfeit his own life by the magistrates, he hastily gave up the boy to his father.

" The Chinese," says Dr. Mackenzie, " expect instant cures. When old-standing cases of disease arrive, and we advise their remaining in the wards, the almost invariable query is, ' How many days will it be before I get quite well?' "

As an illustration of some of the difficulties attending medical treatment, he relates the case of a man who was received into the hospital with fracture of the thigh bone. It had been repeatedly explained to him that he must on no account remove the splint and appliances, and that time would be required to effect a complete cure ; but at the end of a week, seeing no manifest improvement, his friends removed the bandages and splint, and carried him off.

Writing to a friend with reference to the year 1876 the Doctor says :—

" I have been led gradually into doing a good deal for opium smokers, without aiming at very great things, yet seeking to aid those who are enslaved by the terrible drug. Our patients in this department have so increased that we now hardly know where to sleep them. As they, for the most part, come from long distances, and support themselves while in the hospital, we feel it to be wrong to refuse them admittance, since they carry to their homes a knowledge of the truth as it is in Jesus.

" I have been much attracted to Moody's work in America in connection with drunkards. There he is finding the gospel of salvation capable of meeting their condition, and in like manner, in connection with these opium smokers, we are looking for some results by presenting to them the Jesus of the Bible as the great remedy for their case. Oh ! do pray for us out here, that we may be kept very near to the great Saviour, to know His methods better, to be filled with His spirit, and to be ever listening to His teachings. I believe it is a living Saviour that these Chinese need ; but I am afraid that the work is hindered by the lack of faith and the want of devotion to His work of some of us workers.

" You will see how the work among opium smokers has been increased when I give you the following figures. I made a rule to treat these cases only in the wards, as giving medicine indiscriminately proved very unsatisfactory. For the first ten months eight persons only agreed to enter the hospital. During the past year the numbers increased to two hundred and thirty-five ; and during the last month and a half three hundred and twenty have entered the wards for treatment."

Writing at a later date, the Doctor states that these cases have continued to increase in numbers, and that in one year seven hundred persons were treated for opium smoking in the wards of the Hankow hospital.

" That a great need," he writes, " has existed for some kindly help to be extended in this direction is very certain. The habit of opium smoking, prolonged for any length of time, plays havoc with a man's natural energy, rendering him indolent and enervated. Few in this condition can, unaided, combat the craving for opium and effectually reform. The attempt is often made, but as often ends in disappointment ; for a time they persevere, but when the intolerable craving, accompanied by extreme bodily depression, with violent aching of the joints and muscular pains, sets in, they fly to their old enemy, and drown themselves in the opium stupor. If the need is being felt in

England for the further extension of homes for
habitual drunkards, much more is the restraint needed
for opium smokers in Eastern lands.

"A large proportion of the slaves of the pipe who
present themselves for treatment come from towns
and villages at varying distances, though many are
residents of Hankow. They come acquainted with our
conditions, and are ready to submit to them. There
is no medicinal specific guaranteed to cure ; the object
aimed at is to relieve the symptoms as they arise,
and so to help the patient back to health and freedom.

"I always tell them the medicine given to them is to
relieve the pain and craving, but they are to pray to
God and believe in Jesus to get the desire taken from
their hearts, and new hearts given to them. They
thus carry back a knowledge of the Gospel north,
south, east, and west.

"It will be asked, But is there evidence that after
they leave the hospital they do not quickly return to
their old habit? Doubtless some do, but we are sure
that many do not. It would be impossible to give an
accurate proportion of permanently successful cases,
but this is known, that new arrivals seeking admission,
in reply to the question, ' What has brought you to
the hospital for treatment ? ' almost invariably answer,
' I have friends and neighbours who have already
been cured here.' "

The Doctor mentions, among others, the following
case of an opium smoker who was cured, and became
a Christian.

" The man's name was Tai ; he was a fortune-teller, of about twenty-five years of age, and appeared at the hospital emaciated and feeble, accompanied by his mother, an old lady over sixty years of age. The watchful care manifested by the mother attracted our attention, and upon enquiry the following facts were elicited.

" The son carried on a thriving business as a fortune-teller, but he had taken to opium smoking, which had led to disastrous results. His earnings were squandered, his health was broken down, and his poor old mother made wretched. In consequence chiefly of the entreaties of the old lady, the man applied for treatment, and his mother asked permission to stay and wait upon him.

" Such a case was at the outset very unpromising. Here was a man yielding to moral compulsion in a matter which required the utmost resolution. Yet this step was the turning-point in the man's career ; not only was his cure most complete, but he became interested in the Gospel, drank in the only sure antidote for his disease, and success in treatment followed as a necessary consequence. Who shall say that the earnest desire, the prayer of the heathen mother groping in her darkness, was not heard and answered by Him who reads all hearts ?

" With the adoption of Christianity our patient felt that he must abandon his former calling. But his aged mother was dependent upon his exertions for her support ; what was to be done ? To meet this difficulty our dispenser, Siau, who is very active in Christian work among the patients, suggested that Tai should set up in business as a dealer in nuts. This having been his own trade before he was employed in the hospital, he was able to give the ex-fortune-teller all the information needed, and he decided to try and earn his living in this way. This man has since carried on his new occupation, which, though less remunerative than his former means of support, has brought to him and his widowed mother happiness and contentment.

"At the church meeting at which this man was formally accepted as a member a friend of his spoke of having visited his home, and of the consistency of his life with his present profession of Christianity. He told us the old mother had said, ' I am delighted that my son has become a Christian, for although he earns less, he brings me home more money than formerly, and our home is now a happy one.'"

Two other patients who had been cured of opium smoking in the hospital were accidentally encountered by Mr. John while on a boat journey some time afterwards. The wind being unfavourable, he failed to reach the town at which he had intended to stay for the night, and consequently was obliged to anchor at a small village,—a collection of houses merely, all of them shops, which had grown up to supply the needs of the boatmen who might find it necessary to anchor there for the night. It was raining fast, and as the place was so small and the hour late, Mr. John did not go ashore, but sent the colporteur with a few books for sale. After a time the man returned, greatly pleased, with the news that he had been most kindly received by two men of the respective names of Ting and Tsung, who had been cured of opium smoking in the hospital.

Mr. John, upon hearing this, landed and sought out the men. On his way to their house the neighbours, seeing a foreigner, remarked, "We know where you are going,—to the house of Tsung, whom you cured of opium smoking." Mr. John found this man had removed from his house all idols and other relics of idolatry, and both of the ex-patients professed to believe in Christ, and to worship God. Mr. John invited them on board the boat for further instruction that evening. They seemed grateful for the relief given to them at the hospital, and next morning Ting sent a present of eggs on board.

A man from Mien Yang, one hundred miles from Hankow, returned, two months after he had left the hospital, cured of opium smoking. He travelled the long distance a second time in order that he might be baptized.

A barber, who earned one hundred and fifty cash a day, spent one hundred and twenty on opium; as a consequence, want of nourishing food aided the ill effects of years of opium smoking, and brought him into a state of great misery. He heard the Gospel at the city chapel, and, at the request of Mr. John, entered the hospital. He suffered severely for some days, but in the strength of God gained the victory over his besetting sin, and went out healed. He has since been a changed man, invigorated in constitution, and bright and happy in demeanour. Through his earnest activity, but more than all on account of his changed life, others have been won into the Church. One man had kept an opium den and been an opium smoker for fifteen years. He was enabled to give it up and become a Christian. These men are examples of the power of Divine grace. A Tauist and two Buddhist priests were treated for opium smoking at the same time. The hospital assistant referred to this fact at a recent church meeting, concluding his remarks by saying, " How true it is that Jesus is the only Saviour."

" It is very cheering," continues the Doctor, " to see the active interest the native Christians take in the hospital. Many of the Hankow converts are earnest workers for Christ, and when engaged in seeking the conversion of their relatives and friends they often bring them when sick to the dispensary, hoping that the benefits they will get to their bodies, and the kind treatment they will personally receive, may win from them a better attention to and deeper interest in the gospel. One earnest Christian named Koh recently said, when a friend of his was baptized, ' I have brought ten friends, but after being cured, like the lepers in the Gospel, only one has returned to give thanks.' One man was under treatment for a contusion, the result of a beating he had received from his friends because he had become a Christian. Another man of the name of Yang was in the hospital for pneumonia of one lung, from which he made a good recovery. Coming constantly under the influence of Siau, the hospital preacher, he was converted to Christianity, and has since himself been a zealous missionary, having brought his aged father and other friends and fellow-workmen into the Church."

In a home letter, written at about this time, Dr. Mackenzie says :—

" I am beginning to be known at considerable distances from Hankow, for our patients come from far-off places. Mr. Hayt, of the American Episcopal Mission, has been on a journey down the Yang-tse, and upon his return he called upon me. He tells me that many people are enquiring after ' Mah E-Seng ' (my Chinese name); some of them have been patients in the hospital, others are thinking of travelling up to Hankow for treatment. It is pleasant to hear this, because these people would be well inclined to any foreigner they might meet now, and would treat missionaries well after being well cared for in our wards. I have been fortunate in getting a good Chinese name, for the Chinese look very much at the meaning of names. My surname is 'Mah,' the sound that the Chinese would give in trying to say Mac. My second name is ' Kun-ge,' which means that my kun or root is ge, which means to succour or relieve suffering. As the root is the most important part of a tree, the Chinese say the object of a man's life is his

8

root. So 'Ma-kun-ge,' which is almost exactly as the natives would pronounce the name Mackenzie, means that the 'Kun' of 'Mah' is 'ge,' to relieve people.

"Shun, Mr. John's old teacher, thought of 'Kun;' Mr. John himself of 'ge.' 'E-Seng' is the title given to doctors here."

On April 3rd, 1876, there is a note in the Doctor's diary to the effect that at this time he commenced a prayer-meeting for the in-patients in the evening.

In the middle of the summer Mr. John, with his young colleague, taking advantage of a slight break in the great heat, paid a visit to a place called Hwang-chin-kow, on the river Han.

"We had been there several times during the winter," writes Dr. Mackenzie, "when there was only one Christian living there, and now there are twelve; quite a little Church. These Christians usually come down to Hankow for worship every Sunday, but it is a long way for them; so when the weather is good Mr. John tries to get a service there, by sending one of the native Christians from the older Church to preach to the little band of believers. In the very hot weather, such as we have been having, it would not be safe for a foreigner to go.

"We left about three o'clock on Saturday afternoon, after I had got through my out-patients, in a closed boat, kindly lent by one of the hongs. When we anchored for the night we were some miles up the Han, having had a favourable wind; indeed we were close to our destination. We found it a great comfort to be able to sleep without our mosquito nets, which we had brought with us, for there was a good strong breeze blowing on the river, which kept the troublesome insects away. We had a service with the converts about seven o'clock on Sunday morning in one of their houses, and I very much enjoyed it. I am getting to understand the preacher now, and find it a great treat to be able to follow the sermons somewhat. A man was brought to us at this place suffering from tetanus. After the service, having a good wind, we went on to Tsai-tien, a town of twenty thousand inhabitants; and Mr. John preached for about three hours in different parts." [At this place we find from his diary, what is not mentioned in his home letter, that the missionaries were very badly received; they were stoned several times, and found the people exceedingly insolent.] "The wind was dead against us coming back, and we had to crawl along by constant tacking. As there was no hope of getting our big boat home that night, we called a sanpan, or small boat, just wide enough for us to sit alongside of one another in, and in which, as Mr. John said, it would not do for us to quarrel. We reached Hankow about ten o'clock.

"A patient was brought to the hospital to-day with choleraic diarrhœa, carried on a sort of bed like a small four-poster; he came from a place more than six miles away, and was very, very ill."

In the autumn of 1876 the Doctor writes to his brother :—

"You have probably heard, even as I am writing, that peace has been happily settled with China.

"Sir Thomas Wade, whatever has been surmised in the past, has evidently done his work well. Without the cost of any money, or the loss of a single man in battle, he has obtained everything he demanded.

"New ports are to be thrown open on the coast and on the Yang-tse. There is to be a traffic route from Yunnan (in the heart of China) into Burmah, and a heavy indemnity is to be paid to the friends of Mr. Margary. But what is more important, as likely to create a moral effect on the Chinese nation, is that an ambassador is to be sent to England to apologise to the Queen, and the whole affair is to be published in the *Peking Gazette.*

"It remains now for Sir Thomas Wade to see that these important items are carried out effectively. If this is done it will be a great blow to the Chinese. Such is the ignorance, prejudice, and falsehood to be found in Chinese life, especially official life, that it was the general opinion in the empire that the time had come to drive all foreigners out of the country, and that the sooner war took place the better, as the Chinese must be victorious. When Li Hung Chang went down to Chefoo to arrange matters with our government, it was currently reported that he had gone to order our minister out of the country and declare war.

"On Tuesday last I returned from another trip up the Han with Mr. John. The Han is a small river in China, but would be considered a very important one in England. We went one hundred and twenty miles up it. The banks are very thickly peopled; you are unable to find many hundred yards of land free from villages, and large towns are quite numerous. We went the whole length of our journey before we commenced any missionary work, intending to visit the towns on our homeward journey. We took long walks ashore, and I saw for the first time the cotton plant, which was planted over many acres. Here the plant is not higher than a gooseberry bush, and the little bunches of white cotton hanging among the green leaves on the bushes look very pretty.

" There were also many acres of millet everywhere to be seen, giving a very tropical appearance to the country. The ear of millet grows at the top of a stalk ten and twelve feet high; the very poorest people eat it in place of rice. They cultivate the hemp plant largely also, from the grain of which they express oil, used for burning in native lamps and for mixing with their food.

" The breeding of silkworms is extensively carried on, and there were a large number of mulberry trees. And what was of much interest, I saw the tallow tree, though it was not in fruit. The Chinese use this vegetable tallow largely in making their candles. The berries on the tree, when fully ripe, cast off their outer shell, leaving exposed a white surface, the layer of tallow surrounding the small kernel. We went over one of the numerous manufactories for expressing oil, and saw the whole process. The machinery, as you may imagine, is very rough.

" We commenced work at a large market town at the end of our journey, to which but few foreigners have ever been. The people here have the name of being noisy, and they did not improve their character, as they did their very best to insult us. They are very cowardly, and when they throw at you it is always from behind. However, this was the worst reception we had on the journey, as we found the people less rough in other places. I commenced preaching in Chinese on this trip, which I look upon as a great advance. Mr. John does not know what it means to be afraid, I think. When we entered the crowded streets of a city or town, after choosing a suitable place to preach from, he would tell me to go on into the town and do my best at preaching and selling books in some other part. Of course I went, looking to God to take care of me ; and though at first, when surrounded by great crowds, I was inclined to feel shaky, it soon passed away, and I was much helped in doing my best at preaching, and generally got the people to listen attentively. I was thus able to teach some elementary truths of the gospel.

" The people will tell you, when you ask what they worship, that ' heaven and earth are the greatest, and parents the most honourable.' They will not, as a rule, tell you that they worship idols ; they have no idea of a supreme Being. The people's contempt for foreigners is very great. In walking along the streets selling books and Gospels (we have to charge a small sum for them, or they would be torn up and thrown away) a respectable shop-keeper will call you into his shop, saying he wishes to buy a book. You enter, and he will immediately laugh in your face, saying he wants no books, and make some insulting remark about you.

"This and such-like conduct is occurring constantly while we are in towns, and considering how excessively polite the Chinese are to each other, and how carefully their books exhort to ceremonious and respectful behaviour towards strangers, we can clearly see what is their real feeling towards us.

"This is, therefore, a work which naturally one is very little inclined for ; only when we remember we are working for their benefit, and that our Lord for our good never thought of Himself, we are able to bear such conduct cheerfully.

"Evangelizing in unfrequented populous towns in China gives one a very vivid idea of the life of our Lord while on earth, and the kind of work He must have done ; and especially of the wonderful patience, forbearance, and love He showed when in contact with ignorance, prejudice, and vice. To be serving such a Master in such a cause ennobles every work.

"We lived on native food, and I can assure you enjoyed, on returning to the boat after our excursions on shore, our bowl of rice, with pork, fish, or vegetables, and soon got to use our chopsticks with as much ease and pleasure as if they had been the best Sheffield cutlery.

"This health trip did both Mr. John and myself a

great deal of good, and it was well spent, for we were able to return to our regular work in Hankow with all the more zest.

" During my absence I was able to leave the hospital in the hands of my chief native assistant, Mr. Yang, who is now very competent. I get now and again good practice in surgery. A few weeks ago I operated upon a woman, taking away a tumour the size of a young baby's head, weighing two pounds. She is now quite well. Yesterday I removed a woman's breast for hard cancer, and she is doing well. We have difficulties here which are not experienced at home. I have often to give chloroform myself, and then operate, having no assistants who could be responsible for that, though they are so very useful.

" To-day I took away the right upright portion of the lower jaw of a man suffering from advanced disease of the jaw-bone. I got it away through the mouth after having removed the teeth. He is likely to get quite well, all the diseased bone having been removed.

" My assistant did two operations on the eye to-day for the removal of pterygium. These are growths on the eye very common in China, which almost destroy the sight ; in fact, this man was to all intents and purposes blind. By getting rid of these growths sight is restored.

" I make every serious operation a subject for prayer, and I am thankful to God that no death has occurred after even the most severe operations."

CHAPTER VII.

LIGHTS AND SHADOWS OF MEDICAL MISSION WORK.

CHAPTER VII.

LIGHTS AND SHADOWS OF MEDICAL MISSION WORK.

TOWARDS the end of December 1876 Dr. Mackenzie went down to Shanghai to meet the lady to whom he was betrothed, and whose acquaintance he had first made while they were both engaged in Christian work in Bristol.

Miss Travers arrived early in January, and on the 9th of that month they were married by Dean Butcher in the Cathedral, Shanghai, and left immediately for their station in Hankow.

The hospital continued to grow in popularity, and the Doctor made such progress with the language that he was able, towards the end of the year, to write to a friend, " I preach regularly in the hospital before commencing the out-patients, so that I am getting into working order."

His young wife also began with much enthusiasm the study of Chinese, and when the tea season arrived, and the tea-ships flocked up the broad Yang-tse and anchored over against Hankow, both husband and wife engaged in work among the English sailors in company with Mrs. Griffith John, whose name will be long remembered in the far east as the sailors' friend.

"We are now established in our pretty home," writes the Doctor to his brother, "which looks both thoroughly home-like and comfortable, thanks to Millie's deft fingers."

The daily routine of life was occasionally varied by visits across the Yang-tse to the Wuchang side, or up the Han to the Wesleyan Mission House at the Wu Shen Miau.

It is not possible to give any detailed account of the good work which, with God's blessing, Dr. Mackenzie was able to perform in alleviating suffering in the wards of the Hankow hospital. We select, however, a few cases as specimens of the service which day by day he was enabled to render to the Master, remembering that his one aim all through his career in China was, as he wrote himself, to make medicine the handmaid of the Gospel, seeking, through the administration of medical relief, to advance the cause of our Lord and Master Jesus Christ, thus combining the healing of the body with the curing of the soul, in accordance with the words of Scripture, "And He sent them to preach the kingdom of God, and to heal the sick."

During this year a total of one thousand one hundred and thirty-seven patients were treated in the wards, thirty-three being women; and the large number of eleven thousand eight hundred and fifty-nine out-patients attended at the dispensary.

"The hospital is flourishing more than ever," he writes to his mother; "one hundred and fifteen out-patients one day, and ninety-four the next, all to be seen and attended to pretty well by myself. The in-patients, too, are very numerous; we have forty-two beds, but they are all full, and many lying on the floor; I am having new beds made. Many of the people come from long distances; twenty arrived in one day from the same town."

The Doctor also reports a great increase in surgical work, and rejoices in this, since, speaking generally, and with reference to the purely native medical profession, he gives us to understand that the birthday of surgery has hardly dawned in China, for with the exception of acu-puncture and the lancing of superficial abscesses, operative interference is, as a rule, unknown.

"I am passionately fond of surgery," he writes to his brother, "and never happier than when I am about to undertake some big operation. Can you understand the taste?

"Happily for the Chinaman, fractures are not common among them, and when they do occur they are left pretty much to take care of themselves. A case of compound fracture of the arm, of many months' standing, came to the hospital; the broken shaft of the bone was protruding two inches through the skin. No attempt had been made to replace it, and the patient had remained exactly as the accident left him. Being a young and healthy man, new bone had formed without much shortening of the arm, and the protruding portion, having separated during the healing process, was loosely lying in the cavity, only needing to be lifted out with the fingers. Yet it would have been allowed to lie undisturbed, in spite of the constant unpleasant discharge, until it had actually fallen out. That it is rare for a native patient to sacrifice a limb, even though it be to save his life, is a well-attested fact. This is specially so where amputation is called for in cases of disease, but when after an accident the operation becomes clearly necessary, the determined opposition to it is remarkable. A case in point has recently been in the wards. A passenger on board the *S.S. Shanghai* was struck down by a bale of cotton, and received a compound fracture of both bones of the right leg. He was admitted into the hospital, and an attempt made to save the limb; this proving to be impossible, amputation was proposed as the only alternative. The man, however, would not consent, preferring, as he said, to die rather than lose one of his limbs.

" Of the tumours removed, many are very large in size, but one in particular, from its unusual dimensions, merits description. The case was that of a young man, twenty-four years of age, a native of Kiangse, who presented himself with an immense solid tumour suspended from the loins, not unlike a large ham in appearance. It measured forty-three inches round; his parents had first noticed a small growth in his eleventh year, and it had been continually enlarging, until now, at the end of thirteen years, it had reached its present enormous bulk. Much shock was experienced immediately after the operation, and for a few days the temperature of the body rose ; but in a month the wound had healed, and the patient, relieved of his encumbrance, looked a sprightly, active young man."

Upon his recovery, in token of gratitude for the relief afforded him, this patient sent the following letter for insertion in a daily paper.

The editor introduced it with the remark that for a foreigner to write to a newspaper expressing his indebtedness to his medical attendant might be considered out of place. The Chinese custom, however, is different, and Dr. Mackenzie will, he is assured, feel grateful at this tribute to the excellence of Western surgery.

" *To the Editor of the ' North China Daily News.'*

" SIR,—There is connected with the London Missionary Society of Hankow a celebrated English Dr. Mackenzie, who has been there many years, is skilled in curing all sorts of maladies, and never receives money from any patients whom he cures. For ten years I, a native of T'-Ming-Chow, in Kiangse, suffered from a tumour in my back. At first I did not mind it, but at length it became as large as a peck, so that I could walk with difficulty, and I was much afraid that it would kill me.

" I had engaged many doctors, but no one could do me good. I was compelled, therefore, to go to Hankow in search of a more skilled doctor. Fortunately a friend of mine, named Kwo Shan-kai, recommended Dr. Mackenzie to me.　Accordingly I went with him to the Doctor's.　He, on inspection, said that the tumour could not be cured without cutting it off with a knife, and added that I had nothing to fear from the cutting.　On October 4th last he gave me some narcotic to take, and immediately, with a knife, cut off the tumour, which was twenty-five pounds in weight. In about twenty days I completely recovered.　As a return to the Doctor, I shall thank you to put this in your paper in order to celebrate his name.　I am, Sir,

"Yours most respectfully,

"HU-TSZE-KOH."

"Faith is a wonderful faculty," writes the Doctor, "and common enough in the world.　Would that it were always wisely directed!　Instances of misdirected faith are plentiful in China, and are constantly coming under the notice of the medical missionary.　Here is a specimen.　One day there came into our dispensary a young man of twenty, with a large excavated wound of the left arm, evidently caused by some cutting instrument.　In reply to our queries he gave the following history.　He had a sick father, ill for many months with dropsy, 'who had suffered many things of many physicians, and was nothing better, but rather grew worse.'　Finally, the relatives, assembled in solemn conclave, decided that the faculty having failed, the only hope for the father lay in the filial instincts of the son.　He, the son, must sacrifice his own flesh to save his father's life.　It is delightfully easy to prompt others to acts of self-sacrifice.　In this case the youth, whether he liked it or not, was immolated upon the altar of filial piety, and had patiently to endure while a piece of flesh was cut out of his left arm ; this was afterwards cooked into a savoury meal, with accompaniments, and administered to the patient as the infallible remedy. Either in spite of the treatment, or in consequence thereof, the unfortunate patient succumbed. Yet even now the faith of the relatives was not disturbed ; the principle was sound, therefore the instrument must be faulty ; the lad was surely lacking in purity of motive—his filial piety must be deficient. And so the poor boy had not only his father's death and a bad arm to grieve over, but was looked askance at by uncles and cousins as a sad instance of filial disobedience ! Truly he merited our sympathy."

At the time of which we write there was not in Hankow or its neighbourhood any foreign medical lady to treat diseases of women, and render to them, in times of special need, that help without which lives are so often sacrificed in China.

But the fame of Dr. Mackenzie had spread through the city, and in cases of extreme need he was not unfrequently summoned to attend women in their own homes.

On not a few occasions he was the means of saving life, if the invalid and her friends were willing that she should submit to treatment ; but more commonly, the Doctor writes, when the trouble has been taken to hasten to such cases of emergency, the patient refuses to accept the proffered help. In the majority of instances the people expect a cure to be effected by examination of the tongue and pulse, and by the swallowing of medicine, which they will take *ad libitum.*

In one case in which relief could have been speedily effected, after having sent for the Doctor in great haste, the patient suddenly took fright and refused all assistance ; she was seconded by her female attendants, and the husband, though he was told that if nothing was done for her it would cost his wife her life, helplessly replied, " She won't have it, she is unwilling—I can't persuade her ; " and one of the women remarked, " She prefers to die."

This is only one among many instances of Chinese regard for foreign medical skill, combined with marked prejudice against active surgical interference on the part of a medical man in attendance on native women.

It was during this year that the first general Conference of missionaries was held in Shanghai. Though himself unable to leave his work in Hankow to attend these gatherings, Dr. Mackenzie was deeply interested in them.

" My wife and I," he writes, " have been delighted with the accounts from Mr. and Mrs. John of the Conference doings, and were very glad to get Mr. John's printed address."

This reference is to the very striking and helpful discourse on " The Holy Spirit in Connection with our Work," delivered at the opening of the Conference.

In his diary, at this time, the Doctor records several cases of Christians who had stood firm under severe persecution, and of others who had been enabled to resist temptation when it came to them in the form of promises of an easier life if conscientious scruples were silenced.

A boatman who was in the hospital last year, suffering from a bad attack of sciatica, became a believer in Jesus, and was baptized before his return home.

" At that time a relative of his offered to take him into his business—he was a seller of incense. This would have saved him from an arduous life, but after consulting with Mr. John he refused the offer on religious grounds solely. He was beaten by his former companions at his village home, but seems to be a very earnest Christian.

" Two men came down recently from a place about five miles from Hwang-ching-kow across the lake. Both of them had been badly beaten on account of Christianity. The son was one mass of bruises—his face literally black and blue, a wound on the scalp, and one deep one on his leg. These were inflicted with a pointed spear. Some desperate fellows had attacked the family on account of their faith, and told them they must be off with their foreign religion to a foreign land. They had beaten the Christian's wife and child, and his old father, over seventy years of age, who was not yet baptized. The old man had been getting gradually to believe in the Gospel, and now he has had a beating on account of it, is anxiously asking to be received into the Church. So much for persecution ; it will doubtless sift the Church, but will always lead to its true prosperity."

Another case from Hwang-ching-kow was that of a man who, at the time of the Doctor's visit to that place, had seemed very proud, full of conceit, and averse to foreigners. His wife became seriously ill, and he then bethought himself of the foreign doctor, and brought her into Hankow for medical treatment. They had to remain in the hospital for several weeks ; during which time they became much interested in the gospel. Later on, the man brought down his old mother, who was suffering from sciatica, for treatment, and during this second visit was baptized upon a profession of faith in Christ.

As an instance of Chinese generosity, Dr. Mackenzie mentions the case of a paralytic beggar ; to explain which it should be stated that in the management of Mission Hospitals in China it has been found absolutely necessary to limit the number of cases supported out of the general funds. He was told that he could not be taken in, as he had no money with which to support himself while under treatment. The other patients, however, hearing of the man's need, clubbed together, and agreed to pay for his food while he remained in the hospital.

Towards the end of the summer a serious explosion occurred at a gunpowder magazine in the neighbouring city of Wuchang, and Dr. Mackenzie's assistance was sought. The roof of the building had been partly carried away by the force of the explosion.

" I was much struck by the inhumanity inherent in the Chinese nature," he writes ; " the people stood around, looking with utter indifference upon the sufferers. They showed no willingness to help, and expressed no sympathy ; would perform no disagreeable office, or put themselves to any trouble."

Some of the sufferers, with terrible burns over face, neck, and extremities, were removed to the Hankow hospital, where their agonizing pain had to be relieved by constant sedatives.

" I have been giving you incidents in connection with the hospital, because I have no news. My life is the same every day—regular work, which is very enjoyable, but not abounding in incident or change. I scarcely hear a single item of English news except medical, so that you must not expect letters of deep interest."

About the same time the Doctor was called in to see a lad in Wuchang who had been bitten by a dog supposed to be mad. The animal had injured five or six persons beside. The child was bitten in the right cheek and hand ; he died of hydrophobia some days after.

Early in the year Dr. Mackenzie had written, in a spirit of deep thankfulness, that all his native assistants in the hospital were earnest workers for Christ. The native preacher, he says, who has the special duty of attending to the spiritual teaching of the patients, is growing daily in suitability for the work. The others also give valuable aid in the religious department,

and even the coolie manifests great delight when
he sees patients show any interest in the gospel
message.

Later on he writes : " I constantly find Lieu, our
hospital cook, supporting the patients who are unable
to help themselves, out of his own pocket while they
are being treated in the hospital.   He was formerly
a carpenter, and, before he became a Christian, a very
lawless evil liver and an opium smoker.   Yet at his
conversion these sins, with every other, were just swept
away.   He is continually bringing his old companions
as patients to the hospital, and will constantly pay
for their support if they are unable to do so, though
he is only a poor man himself."

Towards the end of this year two native Christians
died in the wards of the hospital, both, up to the last
moments of consciousness, witnessing a good confession,
and peacefully falling asleep in Jesus.

The first of these was a man of the name of Wang,
a cloth dealer in Hankow ; he had been a member of
the Church for about a year, and was a very consistent
Christian.   " Once in a church meeting," writes the
Doctor, " he stated what a difference had come over his
home since he became a believer in Jesus.   ' Before
this,' he said, ' whenever I came home there was
quarrelling and unhappiness—no rest at all ; now
all is changed.   My wife is happy and bright, and all
is comfort and peace.' "

He had been suffering from dysentery for two
months, and was in an extremely weak condition when

he applied for admission into the hospital. He improved a little at first, but had a relapse afterwards, and died suddenly.

When he was dying, and unable to speak, our hospital assistant, Lieu, spoke to him very tenderly of his hope in Christ, and asked him if he still had faith that Christ had saved him, and whether he had peace in this knowledge. Wang was unable to answer, but nodded his head in affirmation. Lieu also asked him if he had any fear at all, when he shook his head in the negative ; and so this Chinese Christian died firm in faith and rest in his Saviour.

Another man of the name of Shun, who was also in the hospital with dysentery, died shortly afterwards. Whenever he was asked as to his state of mind he always replied that his heart was at peace, trusting in Jesus. He was told that life and death were in God's hands when his recovery seemed unlikely. "Yes," he replied, "and I only desire that God's will shall be accomplished." The converts cared for him most tenderly, and grieved much over his loss, especially his own intimate friends, many of whom he had been the means of bringing to Jesus, while they looked up to him as a guide, and felt that his consistent life was a helpful example for them.

In a home letter of this period Dr. Mackenzie mentions an interesting and successful operation he had performed on a young man belonging to a wealthy family of tea-growers, living at a considerable distance from Hankow. While in the hospital the lad was visited by his old father and two other relatives, who became much interested in the gospel, and carried away to their far-off home a copy of the Scriptures and several other Christian books. " These wealthier men," the Doctor adds, " are very difficult to reach, as they would not condescend to enter our preaching chapels. May the Spirit of God move those who have in any way come under instruction ! "

He mentions also the case of a man named Lieu-ku-fang of Hwang-ching-kow, who had been in the hospital, and was returning home cured. He had been a Christian for some time, and used constantly to speak of Jesus and His love to his fellow-patients. One among them, an intelligent man, with some knowledge of character, replied to Lieu's words by remarking that the preaching about God was very good, but he did not see how people could be expected to believe in Jesus Christ. To this the Christian Lieu replied that the doctrines of Confucius taught of one true spirit, and spoke of the need of righteousness in men's lives ; but no one knew any-thing about this true spirit, or saw the righteousness exemplified in real life. But Christianity taught that Jesus manifested to us God our Father and Creator, so that we might know Him ; that Jesus lived in this world as our Example, and has sent the Holy Spirit to move and work in our hearts, teaching us to do God's will.

At about this time Dr. Mackenzie was called in to a case of attempted suicide under specially distressing circumstances. The patient was a lad of seventeen, highly endowed with many natural gifts, and full of life and energy. He belonged to a Christian family, and had of late been the cause of much anxiety to his friends by his association with men of bad character. He became deeply involved in difficulties, and not being of a strong constitution, a severe cold which he took led to inflammation of the windpipe. Rendered miserable by his past folly, and feeling wretched on account of present suffering, he attempted to commit suicide by swallowing opium. When the Doctor arrived at his uncle's house, where he lived, in response to an urgent summons, he found him perfectly unconscious, breathing with extreme difficulty, and the pulse very weak and feeble. To ease the difficult breathing, which seems to have been the most serious symptom, Dr. Mackenzie opened the windpipe, and inserted a silver tube, giving immediate relief. The lad remained in a state of unconsciousness for two days, but eventually made a good recovery. At any rate for a time young Shun profited by his serious illness, and a decided improvement in his mode of life followed upon his restoration to health. He afterwards, in token of gratitude, presented the Doctor with a pair of scrolls, upon which was inscribed in picturesque hieroglyphics the donor's indebtedness "to the skilful hand which had brought him back from the gates of death."

This case attracted much attention among the Chinese, who had never seen or heard of this operation before, and it gave them a higher idea than ever of the wonders that could be wrought by foreign surgical skill. Not long after, Dr. Mackenzie was sent for in hot haste to attend a case of opium poisoning, and he was urgently requested to be sure and bring with him the tube for making two mouths!

Writing to his mother in August 1877 the Doctor says :—

"I have just finished reading the Life of Bishop Patteson, the first Missionary Bishop to the Melanesians. What a noble life! You should get the book if you have not already read it ; Foster got it from England, and sent it up to us. It is written by his cousin Charlotte Yonge, a religious writer of some note, and is free from the strong colouring which makes so many religious lives one-sided and untrue. The character of the man and of his work is put before you in his letters, which always breathe such a true Christian humility, and upon the testimony of co-workers. The early life at Eton and Oxford is devoid of interest for me, and made me think I should not enjoy the book ; but once the missionary prospect opens before him, all the many noble features of his character come out into full play, and you see rising up to your view one of the most unselfish heroes of modern Christian days. Beautiful life, lived to the glory of God !

"I have just been attending a class which Mr. John holds for the native assistants and others, to teach a more complete knowledge of the Holy Scriptures.

To-day the subject was 'Our Lord's teaching in regard to prayer;' last week it was 'Our Lord's example in regard to prayer.' These meetings are very enjoyable; we turn from passage to passage—in fact, it is a Bible reading in Chinese. John puts questions upon the points that come up, and the members make remarks as they like, while keeping to the point under discussion. I attended the class with the object of enlarging my vocabulary, which is a very small one, but I now enjoy the meeting for itself as much as any one. I am as fond of hearing a sermon in Chinese as in English, or even more so, though now I have but few opportunities of listening to English preaching. But to go back to the class. John took advantage of the subject being on prayer, to say a few practical things about the length of prayers.

"You know that in all Christian churches all over the world public prayer is made too much of a task. A man prays for nearly a quarter of an hour, and in that time goes nearly all over the world. Moody did a great deal to alter this state of things amongst many earnest men in England and America, but no doubt it prevails still very largely, and, as a consequence, it becomes a deadener to all real enjoyment of prayer-meetings, and is probably a prominent reason why so few prayer-meetings are a success. We want in our meetings to have short, pointed prayers, asking for what we are prepared to receive, and so give opportunity to many to join in supplication ; thus bringing about an interest on the part of many, and utilizing this very valuable means of grace."

In a letter written two months later the Doctor says :—

"Since you heard last from us I have been on a journey of a week to Hiau-kan, the scene of our old troubles. On Friday last, at eight o'clock in the morning, Mr. John and myself left the precincts of Western civilization in a small boat, with two coolies to carry our bedding, and two portmanteaus containing a few articles of clothing, books for sale, and food to support life. We had found on previous visits to Hiau-kan that once you leave the banks of a stream, with towns within easy reach, and strike across country, the food to be obtained is almost uneatable to us foreigners, even though we are bent on roughing it. We had therefore provided our own food. Millie had cooked some corned beef very nicely, and what with bread, butter, puddings, and cakes, we had a splendid supply for a week's journey. What a joy it is to have a dear wife to look after you ! Millie is a splendid housekeeper, and makes the house and surroundings look as pretty as any in the place.

"Well, with a fair wind we made rapid progress, and reached our extreme point by water at 5 p.m. the same day ; a journey, by the way, that sometimes takes two days. As we were going to sleep in our small boat, we avoided the landing-place, and anchored opposite some open land, but were soon found out by a large crowd, and Mr. John preached to them for a short time until it was getting dusk. We then had a meal, and settled ourselves for the night, spreading our bedding at the bottom of the boat under a bamboo cover, open to the air at one end. There was just room to lie side by side, though it was a close fit ! In the morning we landed at six o'clock at the village called Pch-ching-tswei, not marked, I am afraid, even on Keith Johnston's maps. We paid our boatmen, our coolies shouldered our packages, and away we tramped across the open country, enjoying the brisk morning air.

" The paths are all on the top of mud banks, which serve to divide the fields, and at the same time afford passage to travellers. There are no hedges, and the fields in the distance look like one large common. The paths being narrow, you are compelled to walk single file, and so the Chinese can carry out their favourite rule of elders always walking in front of juniors.

" Getting on for nine o'clock we came to a pretty spot on the top of a hill, the grave of a Han-lin, or member of the Imperial Academy, the highest degree to which a scholar attains by examination. There are very few of them, and the honour is considered very great. There is no extensive growth of wood in these parts, though every hamlet has a few trees about the houses to act as a shade in summer.

" This grave we chose as our camping-place for breakfast. It was an oval place, marked out by trees ;

a mound of earth was raised over the grave in the centre of the open space, and in front a large stone tablet recording the rank and doings of the great man, whose birthplace was in one of the adjoining villages. He had been Governor of Chihli Province, a predecessor of the present Chinese statesman, Li Hung Chang.

"Under the shade of the trees, for the sun was now getting strong, we took our meal. The hot water which we purchased from a neighbouring cottage was our only drawback, for besides being thick with mud, it was topped with a coating of grease.

"But when one has had a sharp walk before breakfast he is not inclined to look too closely at his refreshments, so we partook of it all with enjoyment. Having again started, we commenced work, preaching and selling books in the larger villages and small market towns through which we passed. Towards afternoon we reached our destination, the Wei-chia-wan, or village of the Wei family. We found all the converts well and happy. Of course we had no rest till a late hour, from the people coming from other villages to stare at us. So we sat on benches on the village green, and talked to them till we were tired; but they took longer to weary of staring than we did of speaking. Tell Alec if he wants to be the centre of attraction — to see crowds of his fellow-creatures travelling for miles to have the privilege of looking at and being near him—he had better come out to China at once as the simplest way to gain popularity. But I am sadly afraid such popularity won't last long, for after a few days' residence our star began to fade, and we became ordinary mortals after all.

" But one has got first to learn not to mind being stared at. I have got somewhat used to it now, and can eat my meals in perfect comfort under the gaze of many eyes. My only objection is when they come so near as to trouble my olfactory organs.

" The day after our arrival at Wei's village was Sunday, so in the morning we had service. It was not so quiet as we could have wished, since it was quite impossible to keep the curious crowd out of the small room. Mr. John baptized six women and four children, all relatives of the converts."

Many other villages were visited on the next day, and in the evening, the Doctor mentions, a very helpful service was held for the Christians, when Mr. John gave an address on the True Vine. Next day they crossed the country to Wei-chia-wan, preaching all along the way. " Here," writes the Doctor, " we found a family of converts very bright and happy, the old grandfather of seventy-three telling us that Jesus was in his thoughts every moment, and that he was looking forward to going to be with Him. Another family was not so promising ; the head of the house had got into a dispute about some land, and was cherishing a very bitter spirit against all mankind. Another man had long desired to be baptized, but he had been a leader in the getting up of dragon and other processions, and felt it difficult to take the decisive step.

Our arrival induced him to think more earnestly about the hindrances to his public profession of faith in Jesus. He was much moved, and confessed his entire belief in Christ, bringing us, before we left, an image of the Goddess of Mercy, which had been in his family for many generations ; also the kitchen god, and finally the ancestral tablets ; and he and his little son were baptized before the villagers. Next morning we had prayers at 5 a.m. with the Christians before leaving. We had to walk all the way to Peh-ching-tswei, as we could not get a boat nearer.

"We sent our servant on ahead to hire a boat, and he got one for five hundred cash ; but when we arrived the man in charge of the jetty, seeing that we were foreigners, took away the boatman's oar, and tried to hinder him from taking us for less than one thousand cash, in order that he, the official, might get five hundred of it for himself. However, we took possession of the boat, and had our packages put on board, and then asked the man in charge if he still intended to stop the boat, as in that case we should put the responsibility of delaying us upon him. Thereupon he let us go after paying one hundred cash for jetty dues ; that is, twenty cash in the hundred, which is what the natives themselves pay.

"These men in charge of wharves, and such-like so-called respectable people, get their living by 'squeezing.' The so-called gentry in the country live upon their wits, delighting in quarrels, that they may gain thereby. When they have money they go in for opium-smoking and gambling, and soon lose it all. We saw an example of this in Wei's uncle, who was once a rich man. He became an opium-smoker, and is now keeping up an appearance of respectability, though without a cash. He lives by borrowing cash, rice, etc., which he never intends to repay.

"I find that the Chinese spend a large amount of money in worshipping their ancestors; more indeed upon the dead than the living. When a child is ill, or any calamity befalls the family, they enquire the cause of the priests. They are generally told that one of their ancestors is suffering some dreadful punishment, and that it will require a large expenditure to set him free. The state of feeling among the people compels a man to give the money, however much is demanded. Then sometimes in the middle of the ceremony the priests will declare that still something more must be done, or the suffering deceased will go back again into torment. And so they go on, till the priests have extracted all the money they possibly can.

"We did not reach Hankow until after 11 o'clock at night, for on our way we came to an obstruction, which quite prevented our boat from going on. It was a dam of mud and matting, placed right across the stream by the fishermen, so that they might fix their mats to it. We had to have a small portion of it removed by our own men, sufficient to allow our boat to pass through."

Shortly after his return from this journey, on

October 30th, Dr. Mackenzie's heart was gladdened by the birth of a little daughter. The child was baptized by Mr. John at the usual Chinese Sunday service, and was named Margaret Ethel.

The succeeding winter was an unusually severe one in Hankow. Not only was the Han covered with thick ice, but the great Yang-tse itself was frozen over in parts, and one of the large river steamers had to cut a channel for herself in order to reach Hankow.

Famine prevailed in the northern provinces of China, and in Hankow there was also much distress.

" One benevolent society alone," writes the Doctor, " has given out as many as one hundred and forty coffins to bury people found dead in our streets in one day ; and there are many such institutions.

" In consequence of the unusually severe weather some bad cases of frost bite came to the hospital. One young girl of nineteen had lost her toes and the adjacent skin, leaving the bones protruding ; so I amputated her feet, leaving the heels behind, which will give her as good walking power as most Chinese women possess.

" I must tell you now of a fresh experience I have had in Chinese life and customs. On the first day of the Chinese New Year I went with Mr. Bryson to see the ceremony of worshipping the Emperor in Wuchang. This ceremony is gone through by the Viceroy and other high officials, both civil and military, who are holding office. Wuchang is the capital of the

Hupeh province ; so here you get a good opportunity of witnessing this ceremony being carried out.

"We got up at four o'clock in the morning, and started off for the Emperor's temple. During the walk through the streets I was struck more than I had ever been before by the wonderful hold idolatry has upon the mass of the people. The night that ushers in the New Year is spent by the Chinese in worship. Every house is lit up, and crackers are being let off incessantly, making the night hideous as you walk along the dark narrow streets. Through the open doors we could see incense and candles burning before the family god and ancestral tablet. The worship of heaven and earth we had many opportunities of seeing. A man would come into the street with a small wooden or clay stand, with five holes in it ; in the three centre he places sticks of incense, and in the outer ones candles. These being ignited, he places the stand in the middle of the street before his door. He then proceeds to set fire to some paper money, which he throws burning into the air. A straw mat is then brought out, and he kneels down upon it, facing the incense and candles, and knocks his head against the ground ; this he repeats about five times, and then gets up. His sons, according to age, then follow his example, and after letting off crackers they go into the house. Within doors there is ancestral worship and the worship of the family gods to be gone through, and finally the children worship their parents by prostrating themselves several times. On the previous day I had visited the Emperor's temple that I might examine it by daylight, and so understand the ceremony better.

"The temple is a good specimen of Chinese architecture, its exterior making a pretty picture. It is approached through two large stone-paved courtyards, guarded by huge prison-like doors. The inner court, as you near the temple, has three stone platforms rising one above the other. Once in the temple you find a spacious, lofty building, occupied only by a dais and large incense altar ; these are placed opposite the great doors of entrance. The platform has three tiers, ascended by steps, very rickety from age. On the platform is a large arm-chair, or throne I suppose it should be called, with a screen at the back. The remainder of this large hall is perfectly empty. The chair, screen, and dais are all in a terrible state of dilapidation. The Chinese officials take care to spend very little money upon repairs.

"On New Year's morning, before the dawn of day, guided by our lantern, we made our way through the chairs and retainers of the great men, assembled around the temple, to one of the doors, where, hidden by the darkness, we managed to enter. We had feared we might possibly be stopped. Hastening through the outer courtyard, we entered the inner one, and congratulated ourselves upon safely getting through. We were not long, however, before a small mandarin and a soldier in attendance were sent to take charge of us, and see that we did nothing outrageous. They fancy we foreigners are a species of wild man, unguided by the laws of propriety, and may at any moment do something violent. The hall was increased in size by having a mat roof stretching out in front, under which depended a great number and variety of gaudy lanterns. Soon there was a buzz through the crowd, cushions were spread on the ground, and several officials took their places. They were dressed in handsome satin robes, having broad shoulder pieces worked in gold lace, and wore red tasselled hats, surmounted by glass buttons. The civil mandarins occupied one side, and the military officials the other. In the front line, on the east side or place of honour, stood the Viceroy· Soon the act of obeisance began. A master of cere- monies drawled out the word ' K'wei ' (' Kneel '); the band struck up some music, and all fell upon their knees. 'K'ou t'ou!' he cried, and every head was bent low to the ground. The 'K'ou t'ou' was repeated thrice, and then at the word ' Chi ! ' (' Arise ! ') they slowly resumed their erect attitude, and stood amid breathless silence till the word ' K'wei ' was heard again ; and the same profoundly submissive performance is gone through a second and third time, making in all the well-known three kneelings and nine bendings of the head required of every one presented to the Emperor of the Middle Kingdom.

" The clouds were just beginning to break in the east when we left the temple and wended our way home, with the morning star still shining out clear above us."

Later on he writes : " The cholera has broken out in Hankow amongst the natives, and I am therefore getting some experience of the symptoms of this disease, so rarely seen in England, happily for us. The first day my attention was drawn to it three men were brought to me at the hospital, two of whom died in the waiting-room."

As an instance of the strange cases sometimes met with in the midst of dispensary work, Dr. Mackenzie relates the following to his brother :—

" A man came to the hospital the other day from the country in a very miserable-looking state. He was bent down and breathing badly ; he had suffered from asthma for some time, and was making great complaint. We sent him away with his medicine, and some stramonium leaves for smoking. Two days after, he attended among the patients ; when his turn came he grew much excited, and looked a different man altogether. He began by exclaiming, ' Bless God ! there is no doubt He is the true God, for those leaves that I smoked have taken away my asthma. I am not going to worship idols any more ; they are no good, I shall henceforth worship your God.' He continued in this strain for some time. Stramonium acts like a charm in some forms of asthma, and it had no doubt done so in this case. He was at the hospital again to-day, repeating the same thing. When he first came he seemed to have no mental faculties at all, but upon questioning him to-day I found he knew a good deal of the gospel. I am inclined to think, however, that his smoking the leaves has much to do with this sudden interest in the gospel.

"We have been on a visit to the lakes for a few days. I have been rather pulled down in health, and felt I must get a change. The Wu Shen Miau doctor and his wife accompanied us. We hired a boat with two cabins, and as we were able to stand upright in them, did very well. Our crew consisted of three men and a woman. After sailing for a day and a half, we came to scenery that was far beyond our expectations. We had entered a broad expanse of water, surrounded by hills covered with trees. At the foot of several of these hills were beaches of sand, stones, and shells, with large rocks interspersed about. We could almost fancy ourselves at an English watering-place, with the sea beating upon the beach.

"We spent the days in wandering about the hills and beaches. Little Maggie enjoyed it finely. One especial luxury, too, was to find the population here very sparse—only a few cottages dotted about. So we were able to wander for miles without crowds following at our heels, even though there were ladies with us. The trip did us all good, and we returned to Hankow invigorated."

CHAPTER VIII.

CHANGES—A NORTHERN HOME.

CHAPTER VIII.

CHANGES—A NORTHERN HOME.

WE have seen how flourishing and full of promise was the work to which the Lord had called Dr. Mackenzie in Hankow, and how blessed were its results, both physically and spiritually; so that to most eyes it seemed as if a future of happy and successful labour lay before him in the field which he had chosen.

But God's ways are not as our ways, and not unfrequently we see a man's whole life entirely altered by an apparently inexplicable train of events.

Sometimes, even to the Lord's own children, when such changes come it seems as if there had been some mistake somewhere, as if the Master's will must have been thwarted and His purposes overthrown. And this we are apt to feel more especially when we can put our hands upon some special event, some first link in a chain of circumstances, and say, If that had not taken place this discipline would never have come.

But surely we have allowed our eyes to grow dim

with the mists of earth when we fail to believe that
the loving hand of our Father is leading on through
all the sorrows and mysteries of life, overruling its
heaviest trials for His own far-reaching purposes, and
making all work up smoothly and well into the web
of His providence. Very frequently when changes
come we have to trust, believing simply that what we
know not now we shall know hereafter. Sometimes,
however, God's Fatherly heart allows His perplexed
children to see, even in this world, how He can "turn
life's sore riddle to our good." Not only does He
show us how character is strengthened and purified,
and the heart drawn into closer and brighter communion with its Saviour through fiery trials, but
occasionally even lets us see how His plan of a
man's life is far nobler and higher than ours can
ever be ; how He casts down that He may build up
after a more enduring fashion, and makes even our
disappointments the stepping - stones to higher
service.

And so it was with Dr. Mackenzie, for about this
time circumstances arose, into which it is unadvisable
to enter, which made the Doctor slowly and unwill-
ingly, through painful experiences, come to the conclusion that it would be well for him to seek another
sphere of labour. These circumstances were of a
family rather than a personal nature ; and although
the serious failure of his beloved wife's health, which
shadowed all the later years of his otherwise bright
and successful career, had not as yet manifested

itself, he could not but feel that on her account a change of station was imperative.

Accordingly, he wrote as follows to the Directors of the London Missionary Society :—

"I would respectfully ask you to relieve me of my duties in Hankow, . . . and appoint me to a new field of labour. I believe that while Medical Missions are eminently useful in every stage of the work in China, they would be more than ever successful in pioneering work ; first in gaining the confidence of a strange people, and again in acquiring early personal acquaintance. As the Directors have taken in hand the opening of a mission station in Chung-king-fu, and are seeking men for this field, I beg to offer myself, after three years' study of the language, to go at once and commence work there. I know well what difficulties and privations would have to be endured, while here we have a comfortable home and many friends ; but both Mrs. Mackenzie and I are prepared to face these difficulties."

Some months had necessarily to elapse before the Doctor could receive from the Directors an answer to his request to be transferred to another station. Meanwhile, work in the hospital went on as usual, and 1878 being a year of flood there was much sickness in Hankow, and large crowds attended regularly for relief at the dispensary.

On account of the great lack of surgical knowledge in China, patients will often appear at the dispensary who have been suffering great pain for years, who,

had they come earlier, could easily have been relieved. One case illustrating this fact occurs in Dr.
Mackenzie's diary at this time :—

" A man appeared among the out-patients to-day
with an abscess, which had opened in the palm of his
hand near the wrist.

" Upon examination a foreign body was found lying
close to the bones of the hand. This was cut down
upon and removed, and proved to be a piece of iron
curved and thin. The man explained its presence
there in the following way. Two years ago he was
cleaning out a small cannon, and some powder, having
been left in it, suddenly ignited, discharging this piece
of iron, which was most likely a piece of the gun itself
which had scaled off. It entered the inner side of the
hand, and passing under the tendons lodged there.

" The wound by which it had entered had healed,
and left a prominently marked cicatrix. An abscess
had gradually formed ; but although the man was in
great pain, nearly two years had elapsed before he
came to the hospital and had it removed."

During this summer the floods rose to an unusual
height ; the roads appeared like canals between the
houses, and all communication was carried on by
means of boats ; and the difference between the rise
and fall of the Yang-tse river, seven hundred miles
from its mouth, amounted this season to over fifty feet !

Towards the end of the year Dr. Mackenzie
received a letter from the Directors of the London
Missionary Society appointing him to Tien-tsin.

They felt unable to comply with his request to allow him to proceed to Chung-king and open up work in the province of Sze-chuen, because at that time they did not consider the place safe as a residence for a married man. Soon after this the Doctor received a very cordial invitation from the members of the Peking Committee of the L. M. S. to come and join them, and in addition a private letter from the Rev. Jonathan Lees, the senior member of the Tien-tsin Mission, warmly welcoming the prospect of the additional strength which Dr. Mackenzie would bring to the force of the Mission.

On December 23rd the Doctor wrote to the Directors in London :—

"I thank you, gentlemen, for your resolution giving me permission to transfer my services from Hankow to Tien-tsin.

"The Secretary of the District Committee has already communicated with the North China Committee, and a reply has just been received, in which Mr. Lees, on behalf of the Peking Committee, most kindly welcomes us to Tien-tsin. I gladly accept this invitation, and will leave for the north at the first opportunity. With the resolution passed by the Board I am perfectly satisfied, and will do my best in my new sphere to throw myself as actively into work as I have done here."

But Tien-tsin, the port of the capital, is entirely closed to trade during the winter season, being blocked up with a solid wall of ice for three months of the year. It was necessary, therefore, for Dr. Mackenzie to delay his departure from Hankow till the beginning of March, by which time steamers would soon be leaving Shanghai for the northern port.

During this winter, in the midst of his active labours, Dr. Mackenzie interested himself in the study of Chinese history, especially with reference to the rise and progress of Roman Catholicism in this great land. The story of the earnest labours of the early missionaries of the Romish Church seems to have had a great attraction for him.

The last days of their sojourn in Central China were spent by the Doctor, his wife, and little daughter on the Wuchang side of the river. Dr. Mackenzie had endeared himself so much, not only to the Chinese, but to a large band of missionary friends, that the parting could not help but be a sorrowful one ; yet all believed that an unseen Hand was leading him onward, although he was leaving a work which, under his care, had been so greatly prospered, for a comparatively new and untried field of labour, as far as foreign medical work was concerned.

It was in the midst of a heavy downpour of rain that Dr. and Mrs. Mackenzie, with little Maggie, crossed the broad Yang-tse for the last time to go on board the Shanghai steamer, which lay anchored at the Hankow bund. A large company of native Christians, as well as many of their foreign friends, had assembled, notwithstanding the incessant rain, to see them on board and bid them Godspeed on their journey. The assistants from the hospital were there, with farewell presents of scrolls, recording the Doctor's virtues and their grief at losing him. "Our parting was quite a trying one," he writes ; "one is much drawn out towards these dear native brethren."

The steamer left Hankow at daybreak next morning, and in his diary Dr. Mackenzie gives some account of their journey down the river.

" Bishop Schereschewsky is a fellow-traveller with us. He has been visiting the American Episcopal Mission in Wuchang after his return from Europe. He has done a great work in China in translating the Old Testament into Chinese. He is a great Hebrew scholar. At breakfast he was telling us of his visit up the Yang-tse eighteen years ago with Blakiston's party. He considers the population of China to have been very greatly exaggerated ; instead of four hundred millions, he would say one hundred and fifty millions. He would call all the different dialects of China one language, excepting, perhaps, that of Amoy. He speaks highly of Tien-tsin.

" We have, as another fellow-passenger, a mandarin, who is a Salt Commissioner, with a retinue of twenty servants. He has a wife with him, with two female attendants. The wife is only No. 3, however ; she is a pretty woman, decked out with jewellery. Like ourselves, he is on his way to Tien-tsin.

" We arrived at Shanghai at mid-day on Friday, 6th March. All the steamers for the north have already started, and not a solitary one remains. However, the faster ones will be returning shortly, so that our detention will not be long. We found Mr. Muirhead and Mr. Taylor living together, both the ladies having had to return to England on account of ill health. Dr. Johnston received us with much kindness, and invited a large party of friends to meet us. The next evening was spent with Mr. Palmer of the Union Church, and we took tiffin with Mr. Laisun.

" The *Pau-tah* steamer came in at noon, and was advertised to leave the same night, and we took passage on her, and I have been very busy getting all our numerous packages on board.

" We had a most delightful voyage. The *Pau-tah* has small passenger accommodation, but Captain Patteson, by his great kindness, made the voyage altogether enjoyable. We had sent back our amah from Shanghai, so we had baby on our hands entirely ; but the captain has children of his own, and loves little ones, and he nursed and played with Maggie finely, so that the little darling got quite to love him, and sat by his side at table at each meal as sedately as possible. It was fortunate we missed the first rush of steamers, or else we should have had a terrible time. The wind, it seems, was so high that the waves were beating over the decks, and it was so cold that the water froze immediately, and left the decks covered with ice. They met large masses of ice in the Gulf, and four of the steamers, coming in contact with them, received such damage that they had to go into dock. They were, moreover, detained eight days at Taku

Bar, and finally had to cut their way through the ice. Yet on this second trip not a piece of ice was to be seen; all was spring-like.

"The *Pau-tah* stayed at Chefoo for an hour, so I went on shore, and saw Dr. Brereton's hospital, and had a hurried view of the place itself. What a magnificent harbour! But the land side is locked in by a chain of hills from much communication with the interior.

"We reached Taku Bar on the morning of the 12th, but had to wait for the evening tide before crossing. We were anchored close to the scene of an accident which had taken place a few days previously. An old P. and O. ship, the *Aden*, used as a cargo hulk, had been anchored there. While unloading into cargo lighters the Chinese had carelessly taken goods from the lower decks, while the upper decks were still full; the consequence was the *Aden* toppled over, and fifty-one Chinese coolies were drowned.

"Taku, famous for its forts, and the scene of two severe engagements with the Chinese, is situated at the entrance of the Pei-ho, the river leading up to Tien-tsin, and on to within a few miles of the capital. Outside Taku is a bar of sand, and we had to shift a good deal of our cargo into lighters before we could cross over at high water. We passed the spot where two English gunboats, having got too near the forts, were riddled by the fire from them, and disabled before they could retire. Our captain told us that when one of the English gunboats aws lying thus at

the mercy of the heavy fire from the Chinese forts,
and losing men in great numbers, an American
captain lying outside, unable to stand the sight any
longer, exclaiming, 'Blood is thicker than water!'
steamed up to the disabled craft, and receiving the
fire of the fort upon herself, towed our boat out of
range.   The walls of the two large forts guarding the
mouth of the river are only made of mud bricks, but
they are said to possess a good many Krupp guns.
The Pei-ho is a streamlet by the side of our old friend
the Yang-tse, only just permitting two steamers to
pass one another; and its seven awkward bends before
reaching Tien-tsin make the distance by water very
long.

"How ugly the mud hovels on the banks look!
Not that they are worse than those in Hankow, but so
much more prominent.   Tien-tsin has much of the
desert about it in appearance—grey and sandy.   Not
a blade of grass to be seen anywhere at this season!

"The weather in Tien-tsin at the present time is very
delightful, bracing and vigour-giving.   They evidently
get the heat much later here than on the Yang-tse,
and I hope and trust milder, for in Hankow it was
hot when we left in March.   I had got to actually
dread the Hankow summers; I think four in succession
were quite enough.   The missionaries here all live
together outside the foreign concession; the London
Mission compound is the nearest to the city.   The
compound is extensive, with two Mission houses
facing the south, separated one from the other by a

small building used as a college for the training of native students. The houses are pretty much alike. With ours we are perfectly satisfied, the accommodation being both sufficient and comfortable. There is a graveyard at the back of the Mission compound, which is a decided drawback, and the smells coming from the direction of the native city are very disagreeable.

"We had a very warm reception from Mr. and Mrs. Lees, with whom we are staying till settled; they have one little girl with them, the other children are at home. Our little darling, whose photograph, I hope was finally received, is now running about the house bravely, and keeping in capital health."

In his diary the Doctor writes :—

" I walked into the city to the native service conducted in the hospital chapel; Mr. Lees preached, the attendance was small. The singing in this church is remarkably good ; I have heard nothing in China to equal it. The tunes of Sankey and Bliss are sung here as heartily and almost as well as amongst foreigners, which is due chiefly to Mr. Lees having a first-rate voice for leading singing. Afternoon service was held in the students' chapel. We have Chinese prayers every morning at nine o'clock."

Shortly after Dr. Mackenzie's arrival in Tien-tsin the annual meetings of the District Committee of the London Missionary Society were held in Peking. The Doctor gives the following account of his visit to the capital :—

" We started on our journey at 9 a.m., and it took us two and a half days' cart travelling to reach Peking, a distance of eighty miles. These carts are heavy, ugly, wooden contrivances, so small that only one person can conveniently sit or lie inside, for there is no seat except the floor of the cart. If, therefore, two persons travel together one has to sit on one shaft in front, while the driver occupies the other. The cart wheels are of great thickness, iron-bound, and very strongly made ; an essential condition for travelling on these bad roads. The axle-tree extends fully a foot on each side beyond the cart, so that in meeting these carts you have to be careful not to come in contact with this protruding axle-tree. The interior of a cart is about five and a half feet long by three and a half feet broad, and the covered part is three and a half feet high. Having no springs, and the road being frightfully cut up with ruts, the jolting is simply awful. We line the interior with our bedding and pillows, thus making a soft cushion to lie upon ; but to prevent your coming in contact with the sides of the cart you have to seize hold of the structure of the vehicle itself to prevent incessant concussions. The soil is impregnated with soda in such quantities that it is a dusty, grey, soft substance, in dry weather easily cut into ruts, and carried about by the wind. Therefore, when a slight wind is blowing you are soon completely covered with dust, which penetrates your clothes and gets into your nostrils and throat. In wet weather the roads are pretty nearly impassable ;

you are ploughing through mud, and getting stuck every few minutes.

"We slept on the way at native inns on brick beds called kangs; these kangs have flues running under them. In the winter fires are lit, and the heated smoke and air travel through these flues, and thus heat it, giving you at least a warm bed to lie upon.

"In approaching the walls of Peking one sees an immense and very strongly-built square tower at one angle of the wall, pierced with numberless openings, in which apparently cannon are placed, ready to open upon any venturesome foe. The cannon, upon further approach, prove to be merely painted boards. It is said that when the allied troops neared Peking they were in a great funk lest they should be cut to pieces by these imaginary guns.

"The streets of Peking are exactly the reverse of those in the south; they are as wide as Old Market Street in Bristol. The people pay a great deal of attention to the frontage of the shops, the carving and gilding being especially fine. Peking is divided into three cities, each surrounded by its own walls and gates. The Imperial city contains the palaces of the Emperor, his wives, and household. None but those in attendance, or belonging to the household, are allowed to remain within the walls, and no strangers are upon any pretext admitted within the gates.

"Then there is the Tartar, or Manchu city, in which the Manchus reside. No Chinese are supposed to reside in it, though of late years many have succeeded in obtaining dwellings there. You know the reigning dynasty is Manchu ; consequently all of this race are privileged, and receive small pensions. They have degenerated, as would naturally be expected, and are now a lazy set of men. Had the Chinese much political ambition they could easily, by combination, throw off the Manchu yoke.

"Then there is lastly the Chinese city, in which most of the trade is carried on.

"The whole week was pretty well taken up with meetings twice a day. Saturday was free, however, so we devoted it to seeing some of the sights of Peking.

"The Temple of Heaven, probably *the* sight of China, occupied the morning, and was a great treat. We got into the first enclosure over the wall ; this is an immense park-like place, covered with grass and wild flowers, and interspersed are groves of fine trees. Within the third enclosure is the covered altar, with its great dome, which is finely carved and painted.

"We were fortunate in gaining admission to the ' hau-tien,' a building behind the covered altar containing the tablet. This tablet is contained in a richly-carved cabinet, the door of which being removed, and curtains of silk drawn, revealed the inscription, four characters in gold on a plain black ground, ' Hwang Tien Shang-Ti ' (' The Supreme Being of the Imperial Heavens '). No idol is to be seen in any of the buildings in this temple. We saw the slaughter-house, with its floor covered with hair, and the porcelain kiln for burning the sacrifices.

" The same afternoon we visited the Lama Temple, which is said to have 1,500 priests in residence. The great Buddha here is ninety feet in height, a huge gilded monster, thirty-six feet broad. A lotus plant is growing out of its arm, and there are 10,000 small images of Buddha in little niches round the gallery.

" We also saw the praying machine, in which the classics revolve and prayers are gone through. At the Confucian Temple we saw two drums, nearly three thousand years old, covered with poetry in the old seal character. They belong to the Chan dynasty, and are as old as the Moabite stone.

" We went also to the Wan Shen Shan, or Hill of Longevity, covered with temples, pagodas, etc., in ruins ; they were destroyed at the same time as the Summer Palace by the British troops. The Summer Palace, which we visited, is in a lamentable state of ruin. Destruction has gone on with rapid strides far beyond the mischief done by the foreign troops. The Chinese, despite the protection of a high wall, enter and pull down fine masses of marble and stone for the sake of getting the pieces of iron which bind these masses together."

Writing to a friend of different aspects of Mission work in Peking the Doctor says :—

" At Peking there are several Sunday-schools, but from what I could see they do not succeed in getting the children of converts. Those who have boarding-schools of course find it easy to take the children in classes on the Sunday. One very capital idea, I think, is that in all the Missions the International Sunday-school lessons are used after translation by a committee ; they go through the regular series.

"We started in carts for Tung-chow on our return journey on May 1st, at which place we took boats, and left immediately for Tien-tsin. We reached home at eleven o'clock at night on Saturday the 3rd, having taken to carts again and made a forced march, in order to be in by Sunday."

CHAPTER IX.

THE POWER OF PRAYER.

CHAPTER IX.

THE POWER OF PRAYER.

WHEN Dr. Mackenzie reached Tien-tsin the prospect, from a Medical Mission point of view, looked by no means bright.

In the year 1860 the surgeons attached to the British forces quartered in that city had conducted an hospital for native practice, which was the means of extensive usefulness. On the departure of the troops, however, the institution which they had originated was closed, and though several attempts were made to supply its place, nothing was in reality effected till the year 1869.

At that time Mr. Lees was enabled, by the kind contributions of the Tien-tsin foreign community, to rent a house in one of the principal thoroughfares of the city, and engage a native dispenser from the Peking hospital to take charge of it.

Much good work was done during the ten years that elapsed before Dr. Mackenzie's arrival in Tien-tsin Mr. Pai, the Chinese dispenser, was a Christian, and a man who had gained considerable practical acquaintance with disease and its treatment under Dr. Dudgeon of Peking, prior to his taking charge of the Tien-tsin hospital, and from time to time Dr. Frazer willingly rendered valuable help.

But when Dr. Mackenzie reached this station he found the institution destitute of funds for carrying on its benevolent work. In a letter to a friend he describes the state of things.

" Mr. Pai had no money to buy foreign drugs, and was treating his patients pretty much after the native fashion. In the January previous to our arrival Mr. Lees had made a collection, the usual annual one among the foreign residents in aid of the dispensary. But the amount of contributions received failed to pay off the outstanding debt up to the end of 1878, leaving the expenses for 1879 and this balance from 1878 still unmet. Such was the state of things when I arrived in March—no money and no foreign drugs. At our Committee meeting held in Peking at the end of April, a resolution was passed asking the Directors to grant me money for drugs ; but this supply could not reach me for at least five months. What was I to do in the interval ? The first thing was to set to work at the language, and pass my third examination ; this I did in May last. But though I could help in the directly evangelistic work of the Mission, I felt as if my vocation was neglected unless I was engaged in some medical practice. We prayed much about it—not ourselves alone, but Mr. Lees and other brethren. It was a time of great spiritual blessing to me personally ; I was brought to feel that there was no help in man, but that God would open a way.

"In thinking over many plans, it was suggested, I believe by my dear friend Mr. Lees, that we should draw up a petition to the Viceroy, setting forth the advantages of establishing an hospital for the benefit of the Chinese, telling him what had been done elsewhere in medical missionary enterprise, and soliciting his aid.

"We hoped that by clearly showing him the terribly neglected state of the city, with its numerous accidents and prevalent sicknesses, we might move him, or rather God might move him, and incline his heart to help us with funds."

A memorial was drawn up in Chinese, and through the courtesy of a consular friend, W. N. Pethick, Esq., was presented directly to the Viceroy, with many kindly words of support.

The Viceroy here referred to is His Excellency Li Hung-Chang, the well-known ruler of the metropolitan province, and one of the guardians of the young Emperor while under age.

"It is he who negotiates treaties with foreign powers," writes the Doctor; "he orders ironclads from England and Krupp's heavy guns from Germany. He has almost despotic power in the enormous region which he governs, and is looked upon as one of the most astute and enlightened of Chinese statesmen, as he is the most powerful, and at the present time is the hope of the party of progress."

The memorial was sent in to this statesman about the middle of May, but was set aside with the brief comment that the object was a very good one and he would consider it.

On July 31st Dr. Mackenzie makes the following entry in his diary: " The last two months have been a time of great anxiety, expecting and hoping, but getting no answer from the yamen. It has been a great time of waiting upon God."

In a letter to a friend he says: " June passed away and July came to a close, and yet not a word of reply came from the Viceroy, until we began to think that truly the matter had been shelved and we were to hear nothing more about it. We were more than ever thrown back upon God. I had meanwhile commenced to attend at the dispensary and dispense a few foreign drugs, obtained at our own cost from Shanghai; but very few patients came. I never had more than twenty in a day. Why I hardly know, except the general belief of foreigners that the Tien-tsin people are so anti-foreign."

This time of suspense was fruitful in another direction. In July the Doctor writes :—

"During the last few months I have spent much time in the study of the language; although both at Hankow and Tien-tsin mandarin is spoken, yet the local differences of dialect are very considerable, and the tones especially are upside down. These difficulties, during the few months I have been here, by constant reading with teachers I have, in a measure, overcome ; and, what is of even more value, I have obtained a command of the language which I never had before, small even as at present it is. As a medical missionary in China can do comparatively little without a knowledge of the language, the extra time thus placed at my disposal is invaluable. Since coming here I have read through the 'Great Learning' and the first volume of the 'Analects of Confucius.' I am now reading through, to correct the differences in the tones, the 'Pilgrim's Progress,' as translated by William Burns. It is a splendidly correct and very simple translation into mandarin. How fresh and bright this remarkable book is in its Chinese dress!"

At last the weary time of waiting came to an end. By another reference to what Tennyson calls "those fallen leaves that keep their green, the noble letters of the dead," we find the Doctor thus gratefully relating the story of how God, in His lovingkindness, answered, in a wonderful and totally unexpected fashion, his servants' continued prayers.

"It was August 1st, and the day of our weekly prayer-meeting, when the missionaries and native helpers meet for prayer and consultation. Our subject that morning was the words of our Lord, 'Ask, and it SHALL be given you.' And again we pleaded for an answer to the memorial, and that God would remember our Medical Mission needs. While we were praying the Lord was already answering. That same morning a member of the English Legation, closeted

12

with the Viceroy, observed that he was very sad. On
asking the reason, the reply was, ' My wife is seriously
ill—dying ; the doctors have told me this morning she
cannot live.' ' Well,' said the Englishman, ' why don't
you get the help of the foreign doctors in Tien-tsin ?
they might be able to do something even yet.' At
first the Viceroy objected that it would be quite
impossible for a Chinese lady of rank to be attended
by a foreigner ; but by-and-bye his own good sense,
led by God's Spirit, triumphed, and he sent down
a courier to the foreign settlement for Dr. Irwin
and for me. It was just as our prayer-meeting was
breaking up that the courier arrived with his message.
Here was the answer to our prayers ! "

The doctors, accompanied by Mr. Pethick, rode up
at once to the yamen of the Viceroy. After an interview with His Excellency, who is deeply attached to
his wife, and in her serious illness had practically
suspended all public business, they were conducted
into the inner apartments, and there saw the sick
lady. This, to Western ideas, would be considered a
very natural and ordinary occurrence ; but according
to Chinese notions it was a very extraordinary
proceeding.

"Three years ago," writes Dr. Mackenzie, " while in
Hankow I was called in to attend a sick lady, the
wife of a merchant, but was not allowed to see her
face. A hole was made in a curtain, through which
her arm was protruded, that I might examine her
pulse and so diagnose the disease. In this case we

two foreign doctors had free permission to examine
and question our patient, who was the wife of the
leading Viceroy of the Empire."

They found the lady very ill—in a most critical
condition, and at first do not seem to have been
hopeful of a successful issue.

It was necessary for Dr. Mackenzie to come down
to the settlement for medicines, and upon his return
home he found a number of Christian natives in his
colleague's study, earnestly talking over the wonderful
event of the day. "What chance was there of Lady
Li's recovery?" was the eager enquiry from all; but
the Doctor could give no very hopeful reply. "She is
very ill; I fear there is not much hope," he said, "but
you must just keep on praying."

He returned to his illustrious patient, and remained
in the yamen all night, to enable the Viceroy, whose
anxiety was now somewhat allayed, to get some
needed sleep.

"We were in close attendance, seeing our patient
twice a day for six days," writes the Doctor, "when,
by the mercy of God, the lady was, humanly speaking,
out of danger."

Dr. Mackenzie's colleague well remembers how, on
his return from the yamen, in reply to his interested
enquiries about the case, he replied, "Yes, she is recovering, she will do well now; but it is the result of no
skill of mine, it is just God answering our prayers!"

"It became necessary for the patient's complete
restoration to health," continues the Doctor, "to adopt

a certain line of treatment, which, according to Chinese etiquette, could only be carried out by a lady. We therefore informed the Viceroy that at Peking (two days' journey off) there was an American lady doctor working in connection with the Methodist Episcopal Mission, Miss Howard, M.D., and enquired if there would be any objection to a foreign lady carrying out our suggested treatment. 'None whatever!' was his reply."

That day a special messenger was despatched to invite Miss Dr. Howard to come to Tien-tsin, the Viceroy, at the same time, sending his own steam launch to convey her from Tung-chow.

Apartments within the Chinese palace were prepared for her, and here, upon the lady's arrival, she took up her abode, remaining in the yamen for a month, and was able to render invaluable assistance in the case.

"If you will try and realize the conditions of an Eastern city," writes the Doctor, "you will quickly understand that when a great potentate takes you by the hand the land is all before you.

"So we found that in our daily visits to our noble patient our steps were thronged with eager suppliants, who, hearing that the Viceroy's wife was undergoing medical treatment, sought for relief from the same source. You know how a story often grows as it spreads, and so this case of cure was being magnified into a miracle of healing.

A Chinese official residence is composed of numerous quadrangles, one behind the other, with buildings and gateways surrounding each. To reach the family apartments we had to pass through these numerous courts, and here we were beset with patients from the crowds assembled outside the gates, and the friends of the soldiers, door-keepers, secretaries, and attendants who had succeeded in gaining an entrance. The poor also besieged us as we entered and left the yamen. It was truly a strange gathering we found daily collected round the outer gates—the halt, the blind, and the deaf were all there waiting to be healed; indeed, the whole city seemed to be moved. High officials sought introductions to us through the Viceroy himself.

"We had many opportunities of conversation with the Viceroy and other officials, whom we were daily meeting at the yamen; and I trust our conduct was such as to give them a right impression with regard to missionaries and their work; for certainly, with the exception of His Excellency, who is remarkable among Chinese for his breadth of view and friendly feeling towards foreigners, few seem to understand the purpose and object of the missionary's life.

"One day Dr. Irwin and I proposed that the Viceroy should himself see a surgical operation performed. Upon his consenting, we turned the courtyard in front of his audience chamber into an operating theatre. It is a large open space, surrounded on three sides by buildings, the central one being the grand reception room, where ministers from foreign countries

have their interviews with the Viceroy. On the
fourth side the wall is covered with creeping plants,
while ornamental shrubs in pots are placed about the
yard. Li Hung Chang stood looking on, and surrounding him was a crowd of officials and attendants,
attracted by curiosity. His appearance is that of a
man born to rule ; he is six feet two inches in height,
with a truly commanding figure, and a calm, powerful
face. In the centre of the court was a table, upon
which lay our patient, with a large tumour, the size of
a child's head, growing from the back of his neck.
We administered chloroform and removed the tumour,
of course without the man feeling any pain during
the process.

"Two other cases were also operated upon, one
patient having a hare-lip, the other a malignant
tumour. All these cases did well ; wherein again we
see the hand of God helping us. The effect upon
the Viceroy and officials was marked. It was evident to them that crowds of people were waiting to
be healed, and that in Western medicine there were
possibilities quite beyond the reach of the Chinese
faculty. This led to the Viceroy placing a room
outside the gates of the yamen at my disposal for
dispensary work. Here I saw cases daily, but the
crowds became so great as to impede the business of
the yamen, and therefore His Excellency set apart an
entire quadrangle of the temple to Tseng Kwoh-fan,
one of the finest buildings in Tien-tsin, for dispensary
work, and, if necessary, for the reception of in-patients.

"Shortly after the work had been started in the temple, the Viceroy put up a tablet over the entrance, with his three titles inscribed upon it, and beneath them the words 'Free Hospital.' The Viceroy at the same time handed me tls. 200 to purchase drugs for immediate use, and gave me a commission, appointing me, with Dr. Irwin, medical attendant upon his family and yamen, and a separate authorization to establish and superintend the free hospital at the temple.

"In thus giving me the use of his name and taking upon himself the support of the work, His Excellency knows I am a Christian missionary and will make use of every opportunity for the furtherance of the gospel. An evangelist of Mr. Lees' preaches regularly to the assembled patients."

In another letter Dr. Mackenzie explains the Viceroy's action in supplying him with money to purchase drugs and instruments for the hospital ; and with reference to his appointment as physician to the household of His Excellency, and the question of remuneration for his services, writes : "I requested that if the Viceroy wished to make any return to me he should do it by helping on my Medical Mission work. I therefore receive no salary, but all the cost of the medical work at the temple is borne by His Excellency.

"From the commencement I have been unable to compass the work, so many have applied for treatment. Every help has been given me ; a handsome pony and English saddlery, with ma-fu, have been provided, and a military official comes daily to conduct me to and from the temple, or to the various yamens of the city.

"Mr. Pethick has given great help in getting the mass of work into some order. Every case is now entered upon a separate sheet in a large day book. The number of this page is given to each patient on a ticket, and when he comes again he has to produce it. One very striking feature about this dispensary work is, that the old patients attend so regularly, and from the number of applicants all slight cases are excluded. Thus in a day I may only take on twelve or fourteen new cases, but see over a hundred old cases. As the days have shortened, I now attend at the temple from 10 a.m. to 4 p.m., and on Saturday last saw over two hundred cases; yet many had to go away unseen.

"All the helpers are untrained men. Mr. Pai was too much of a native doctor with a private practice to care to assume a subordinate position for a moderate salary and no private practice, so he has left us, and we have closed the old dispensary. It is much better as it is, for I can train the present staff my own way.

"The opening here for Medical Missions is so remarkable, all classes and both sexes eagerly seeking aid, that after Miss Dr. Howard's return to Peking I wrote to the Committee, with her consent, urging her transfer to Tien-tsin, to take up the splendid opening for work amongst the women here. She has

therefore come down to Tien-tsin with her Chinese
women, and commenced work, taking the female
department at the temple, the entire support of
which is borne by Lady Li.

" Though the temple has ample accommodation to
satisfy the most ambitious for in-patients, the distance, three miles from the Mission compound, made
it very awkward to leave severe cases, especially after
surgical operations, so far off. Had I been alone I
should have taken up my abode in the temple ; but
this was impossible, and would have been very unwise from a health standpoint, besides which it was
very desirable that the in-patients should be more
under the influence of Christian surroundings.

" But our Heavenly Father, who has thus wonderfully answered prayer in giving funds and an open
door to the people of Tien-tsin, can also give us a
permanent hospital."

We see, therefore, that up to this period the Medical
Mission work accomplished in Tien-tsin had been
largely confined to the outdoor department, and as
many as two hundred and fifty sick persons were
often congregated at one time in the large court of
the dispensary.

Dr. Mackenzie was feeling more and more that the
grand work to which he had been called was unsatisfactory, from a medical point of view, for one
foreign physician, single-handed, with untrained native
assistants, to compass. Moreover, although a dispensary gives large opportunities for relieving the

sick, the prospects for doing lasting spiritual work
are not very hopeful.

" A gospel address is always delivered to the waiting
patients, but they are usually so fully occupied with
their own ailments and the novelty of being treated
by a foreign doctor, that they can spare little thought
for the glad news we so much desire to tell them."

It was not wonderful, therefore, that Dr. Mackenzie
earnestly desired to see a hospital erected, since it
would prove so powerful an aid to the evangelistic
work of the Mission, which always lay so near his
heart, and, moreover, was urgently required whenever
serious operations were performed.

It was decided to erect the hospital on a vacant
space of the London Mission compound.   Plans were
drawn up by Mr. Lees and Dr. Mackenzie, and having
been submitted to some of his wealthier patients, he
found them very willing to give out of their abundance
for the relief of other sufferers.

" The patients have shown a readiness to help," he
writes ; " besides presenting tablets, etc., they have
now and again sent subscriptions.   A general came
and lived at the hotel in the concession, in order that
I might attend him for dysentery.   When he was well,
and called to thank me, I told him of our desire to
establish an hospital in our grounds for the reception
of severe cases that could not be left so far away at
the temple.   He wanted to see the plans ; they were
examined, and when he next called he subscribed
tls. 500.

" This general had been very bold in his defence of Buddhism against Christianity during my visits to him, and had uttered some bitter things against our Saviour. I was surprised to find his acquaintance with the Bible very considerable ; yet he was intensely antagonistic. He had been in the Taiping rebellion, and had become acquainted with a mongrel form, if one dare to call it so, of Christianity ; and yet God moved his heart to give thus liberally to aid our plans.

" The Prefect of the city, also a patient, who had established a native dispensary in Tien-tsin some months ago, upon leaving, when promoted to the provincial capital, closed the dispensary and handed over the balance of its funds, tls. 300, to our new hospital account.

" Another official, the Customs Taotai, when I called and laid the matter before him, gave us a subscription of tls. 1,000.

" The subject was mentioned to the Viceroy, who approved of it, and handed me a letter authorizing Mr. Pethick, U.S. Consul in Tien-tsin, and myself to make a public subscription in aid of my work. He also offered himself to subscribe tls. 1,000 ; but as the entire support of the dispensary work was borne by His Excellency, we judged it best not to tax his - generosity too suddenly, but to wait the result of a public appeal."

Before the above-named subscription list was issued, however, through the sums contributed by grateful patients alone Dr. Mackenzie was able to prepare the ground and complete one ward of the hospital.

"This hospital work," he writes, "gives remarkable opportunities for circulating the gospel message through the length and breadth of the land, for already many of the cases have come from long distances, and in every instance have returned with a more or less clear knowledge of gospel truth. As yet we are making the in-patients provide their own food, but are compelled so many times to refuse admission to needy cases, suitable subjects for operation or treatment, that I am hoping God will send us sufficient funds to support a few free beds. To keep a bed occupied all the year round here in China would only cost a five-pound note, and yet be the means of incalculable good to some eight or ten crippled or diseased people, and open up to them such an opportunity of religious teaching as can be obtained in no other way.

"I get numerous opportunities of introducing the subject of Christianity to the highly-educated Chinese, and find that when wisely approached they will listen respectfully and with attention, though ever ready to find parallel truth in the teachings of Confucius.

"The work now is only limited by one's strength and capacity. May God give us strength in our great weakness."

With hands and head constantly occupied with congenial work, and seeing success crowning his efforts on every side, it is scarcely to be wondered at that Dr. Mackenzie taxed his strength to the utmost, till at last the strain became too great, and nature took its revenge.

"I am so tired," is a remark that occurs more than once in the letters written to his mother during the latter months of this year, and the weariness culminated at last in a serious attack of illness.

"Your warm-hearted New Year's letters came safely to hand not many days after the period they were intended for," he writes in a home letter. "They came to brighten us just as I was recovering from a sudden and sharp illness, and was lying prostrate from weakness. It was just another but more severe attack of my old enemy malaria, but complicated by slight congestion of the brain. But God in His mercy would not let it go too far, and I am, though still weak, I trust a wiser and a better man. In such times of affliction there is no comfort or consolation in any other but in our Saviour Jesus. Though my life has been so full of disobedience to that dear Saviour's commands, yet as a sinner solely relying upon His grace He never left me, and I felt His loving strong arms protecting me, even when so seriously ill. I was so happy, and had, oh, such perfect rest. Don't think that I am trying to preach a sermon ; I cannot help writing what I have. Who can comprehend the love of God for sinful men ? It passeth a mother's love. Everybody has been so good and kind to me it makes me marvel, and I bless God for it.

"Mr. Pethick sat up three nights running. Dr.

Irwin, besides being with me three times a day, took what he could of the temple work, with Pethick interpreting. To-day I have had a call from the Governor of Tien-tsin, the Taotai. I treated him formerly for an attack of bronchitis, and so he now came to ask after me. Eastern dignitaries go about in state, and the official retinue in this case extended about a hundred yards up our compound."

On May 11th, 1880, the Doctor writes :—

" The work continues to prosper through the blessing of God. I have my hands full now in the hospital, so I only go up four days in the week to the temple. It is pleasant to see the buildings rising up about us here, within sight of the window as I write. This gives some good guarantee, were one needed, of the permanence of the work. Not that the interest of the Viceroy abates in the matter at all, but some people ask, what would happen were the Viceroy to die or leave Tien-tsin? Such contingencies do not trouble me, as I believe it is God's work, not ours. We are not trusting in the princes of this world, but in the help of the King of kings, who has already started this work, and He will not forsake it, I am sure. We only want to use more our privilege of prayer, through faith in Jesus. It is most marvellous to think that God promises to hear and answer prayer when in the name of Jesus. Especially is this manifest when we are in felt need. Only within the last week the truth of this came strongly home to me. A patient was brought to the hospital in great progress ; he could hardly breathe, and was in an agony of pain. His illness was of such a nature as to necessitate operation as the only chance of recovery. On the evening after operation the patient became almost pulseless. He was besides in great pain, and his friends comforted him by saying he was sure to die. After doing all I could for him, I imitated the men who brought the case of palsy to our Lord to be healed, and laid this man's case before Jesus. He heard my prayers and the prayers of dear Millie, and the next morning there was a very great improvement in the man, since which time he has been daily getting better.

" It would probably be difficult for a medical man in England to comprehend my anxiety over such cases, for you have to be in these circumstances to understand them. At home in such serious cases consultants are called in, and whatever operation is undertaken, be the result what it may, it is accepted that the best thing has been done for the patient. Here I am alone ; Dr. Irwin would come if I sent for him, but I do not like to be troubling him too frequently. Then the Chinese, though they see a man is very ill, don't realize that unless operated upon he must die. If he should die after the operation, they would be sure to spread abroad the news that our operation had killed him, and so the work would be seriously damaged from false reports.

" Since commencing this letter I have had an interview with the Viceroy. He wants me to start a vaccine establishment in connection with the temple work ; so I have agreed, and sent for a supply of vaccine to Shanghai. I must teach some Chinese how to operate, as I have no time to do it myself. I vaccinated the Viceroy's little son, two years old, in the yamen. I saw a young Chinaman to-day just back from Germany, where he has been studying military science ; a most promising young fellow, but come back only to die, as he is in a most rapid consumption, and cannot, humanly speaking, live more than a few weeks."

Shortly after this Dr. Mackenzie writes :—

"It seems to me, with my experience of missions, to be a very foolish thing that the Churches at home who are interested in missionary work do not take up more earnestly the subject of Medical Missions. I believe they find a difficulty in getting men ; but if they were to make a special point of it, they could surely get more, and even, if necessary, they might train men. In a land like China there should be a medical missionary in every station, particularly for pioneer work in the interior. I believe I could go and settle anywhere, acting cautiously and wisely, and be undisturbed by the people ; and so could any medical missionary after some experience. And yet they have a bare handful of qualified men in China in the various Missions.

"My medical work comes so congenially to me with my present hospital for in-patients. I have a splendid field for surgical practice, and it is becoming more and more a passion with me. I love my medical

work for its own sake, and more so still when I know
it is paving the way for blessings yet in store for this
land."

In the summer of 1880 there seemed every prospect
that China would become involved in war with Russia.
Sir Thomas Wade was staying in Tien-tsin for several
weeks, and was holding frequent interviews with the
Viceroy. During the course of this visit Li Hung
Chang gave a banquet in foreign style, inviting six
foreign gentlemen and eight of the principal Chinese
officials to meet the British minister. Drs. Irwin
and Mackenzie, the Viceroy's medical advisers, were
included among the guests.

His Excellency seems to have spoken to Sir
Thomas in the most appreciative terms of the good
work Dr. Mackenzie was carrying on, under his
patronage, for the relief of the sick people of Tien-
tsin, and to have singled him out for special marks
of favour during the banquet.

" I felt thankful to the Viceroy, because I know he
was speaking according to his own judgment," he
writes to his brother. " No foreigners have biassed
him in my favour ; the fact that I am a Missionary
effectually precludes that."

Dr. Mackenzie was perhaps over-sensitive on this
point ; he seems to have taken it a little too much for
granted that the motives which led him to devote his
life to caring for the spiritual as well as the bodily
needs of the Chinese around him could not be appreciated or understood by the majority of his fellow-

countrymen in China. He thought, because he had deliberately set aside all thought of accumulating wealth for himself, there must necessarily be an insinuation of inferiority tinging all their thoughts of him. But whatever the opinion of foreign communities in the East may be of missionaries generally, it is certain that Dr. Mackenzie's professional skill and noble character were held in the highest estimation by all who knew him ; while with regard to religion they viewed him in the light of an enthusiast.

About this time there is a record in the Doctor's diary of an interview he had with General, then Colonel, Gordon, who was staying in Tien-tsin, having come to North China at the request of his old comrade-in-arms, Li Hung Chang, to discuss and advise upon the difficulties in which China was then involved.

" During his stay in Tien-tsin Colonel Gordon was residing in 'our temple,' in the quarters set apart for the guests of the Viceroy. It is very extensive, and has splendid accommodation after Chinese style. Gordon is truly a godly man, of the rare old Puritan type. I was greatly delighted and instructed by his genial conversation. He is a Christian soldier, reminding one of Havelock, and a man of men. He is looking strong and hearty, and has a very pleasing face. Evidently, from his conversation, he is a very earnest student of the Bible, which was lying on the table at his side. He spoke of his own spiritual experience, of his faith that God would not allow him to want, and therefore he felt that he had no right to store up money or give any anxious thought to the future. To strengthen my faith, he informed me that when he left England he gave to his brothers all his money, reserving only £80 for his journey. When he arrived in India he had with him only £9 sterling. When he resigned his post as secretary to the Marquis of Ripon he had only £1. He might have remained at his post for a while, until he received a portion of his salary, which would have tided him over; but feeling it to be his duty to resign he did so, and borrowed a few pounds to meet incidental expenses. The day after came a telegram from Peking, inviting him to come to China; and so the financial difficulty was removed. When he reached Chefoo, in consequence of a letter he received from Sir Robert Hart he thought of turning back, and going again to Egypt. However, he finally decided to come on and see the Viceroy, at any rate. He preferred to sleep on board the steamer the first night, after which he removed to the T'seng-kung-su, so as not to implicate any one.

"He also received instructions from home telling him that his 'leave' was stopped, and that he must return at once. He, however, determined to have an interview with the Viceroy, at which he asked him plainly, 'Do you want me? If you do, I will stay with you. But are you, with your military officers, prepared to effect changes? If not, it is no use my staying. For any good to come of it you must do the work yourselves, and I will help you.' Gordon said he liked the Viceroy very much, and the Chinese people generally, and he thought them very good-hearted. He said, how little foreign merchants in China seemed to know of the Chinese. With reference to the troubles which were the cause of his visit to this country, he remarked that he had told the Viceroy if he was really required he would stay, and help them, if possible, to settle matters quietly. If, however, war was forced upon them, he would fight with them to the last; all he required was a coffin and a hole in the ground. As he was their servant, he should expect to have his expenses met, but he desired no other recompense. He had at once telegraphed home, resigning his commission.

" He said he had learned to say, with Paul, ' I am the chief of sinners,' as an actual experience; that in himself he felt there was no particle of merit, not the slightest thing that he could hold up as worthy of praise. He did not attend church, except in England, for example's sake, for he so rarely heard the gospel, that is, ' Glad Tidings,' preached. He believed in preaching by the life. Clergymen, he said, so often preached, ' Do good, and you will go to heaven ; do evil, and you will go to hell.' For himself, he preferred living with the publicans rather than with the Pharisees. He was weary of this world, and longed for death, which appeared to him to be a much-desired event, leading to the Haven of Rest. He thinks the nobler life will begin in the next world, and is waiting for it.

"While in Africa, in the Soudan, he was a perfect sovereign. He had a box in front of his palace, with a slit in it, and whoever had a grievance could drop a petition into this box, which would be attended to by himself. He spent all his income upon the people, and brought nothing away with him. Since he has been here the Viceroy has sent him presents and money; but he returned everything, except two boxes of tea. He never had any doubts upon religious subjects; 'They were all cleared away now,' he remarked. He is such a bright, happy fellow, he makes everybody love him who comes near him. I was struck with one thing about him, and that was, that religion had become a part of his life. Not that he uses religious phrases; I fancy he has an abomination of cant, or anything approaching to it; but it is natural to him to refer to spiritual things. You can't help recognising the sort of man he is."

It is interesting to read of this interview between these two men, both of them on terms of familiar intercourse with the great Chinese Viceroy. The inspiration of their lives was the same—a simple faith, not only in the unseen and Eternal, but in a living Saviour; and it enabled them, as the graphic translation of the Lutheran Bible has it, to hold on to Him they saw not, as though they saw Him.

It would be strange if the Viceroy, with such types of Christian character as these before him, should not at times have exercised his mind over the faith which influenced them.   Dr. Mackenzie was often questioned as to whether he saw any leaning towards Christianity on the part of those in high places with whom he was constantly associated ; and he was always careful to explain that, even as in the Judea of old, it would be indeed hard for the rich and powerful of this land to receive the religion of Jesus.

With regard to the Viceroy's own feeling on the subject of Christianity, it is well known that on one occasion he expressed, in no measured terms, his surprise that a people so cultured and intelligent as those of the West should, as the very foundation of their faith, give credence to a story so improbable as that of the incarnation of our Lord.   Similar legends were prevalent in the East, he admitted, in connection with other religions ; but none but the common people believed in them.   To the end of Mackenzie's life the Viceroy ever regarded him as a man of noble character and high aims, but at the same time he looked upon him as almost a fanatic with regard to religion.

The Doctor always expressed in the highest terms his admiration for His Excellency's kindness of heart, remarkable administrative ability, and far-reaching views in reference to the immediate and future necessities of his country.

Writing to a friend in England, who had asked his opinion with regard to the treatment of the Chinese in the state of California, Mackenzie says : —

" The Americans have sent a new minister and two special commissioners to China to make a new treaty with reference to emigration and the Californian trouble. Well, they have finished their work, and a few days ago, when the Viceroy was handing the treaty already signed back to the commissioners (for His Excellency is also Grand Secretary of State), he said, 'This treaty has been drawn up in the spirit of Christianity, and it reflects honour on both nations.'"

" Tien-tsin has been upset of late with war rumours," he writes a few weeks later, "and our subscription list for the hospital has been necessarily set aside ; however, the building still goes on, and the roof will shortly be finished. We are wanting about another thousand taels to complete it. If we had matters settled quietly this sum and more could be obtained without much difficulty. In case war comes, I will ask the balance from the Viceroy to complete the building for the reception of wounded soldiers. I have already promised him that in case of war I would accompany him and the troops into action, and do what I could for the wounded."

" We have had such nice guests staying with us, on their way to the interior," he writes in a letter dated November 13th. " Dr. and Mrs. Schofield are great additions to the missionary body in China, and make one realize that the spirit of self-sacrifice is as strong now as ever it was. They have independent means, and have come to China, at their own cost, in connection with the China Inland Mission. He is a man who could hope for the highest position in medicine in London—is an M.D. and M.A. of Oxford, and has been on the staff of St. Bartholomew's Hospital. He has travelled very extensively in America, Palestine, Greece, Turkey, and all the great countries of Europe. He preaches in French, German, and English, and although he has been in China only three months, he already speaks better than most men after a year. He has studied medicine in London, Paris, Berlin, and Vienna, and served as an ambulance surgeon in the Turkish war. Now, with life opening before him, at the age of twenty-nine, he has determined to devote himself to medical missionary work in China. Most people would say he was throwing himself away, and that all his fine education was being wasted. But not so ; he could not have a nobler sphere than to be engaged in the fight to open China to the gospel. He is going into Shan-se to Tai-yuen-fu, and as a medical missionary will be an immense gain to them there. We greatly enjoyed their visit of four days, for he is a splendid fellow, so manly, and yet so humble a Christian."

It was on December 2nd, 1880, that the new hospital, the funds for the building of which had been entirely supplied from Chinese sources, was publicly opened by His Excellency the Viceroy. The occasion was one of such special interest that it elicited the hearty co-operation of both Chinese and foreigners.

In the course of a detailed account of the opening

festivities given by the *North China Daily News*, it remarks :—

"The occasion deserves more than a passing notice. It exhibits a new and important phase in the history of Medical Missions in China. Hitherto the work of these Missions in this country has been carried on almost entirely by foreign aid, the occasional sub-scriptions received from native sources having been very small. Unique interest, therefore, attaches to the work carried on by Dr. Mackenzie during the past fifteen months, seeing that all the funds for its support have been derived from native sources."

The hospital is built on the Taku Road, the principal thoroughfare between the foreign settlement with the shipping and the native city.

The Doctor gives the following description of the building, which, as he always said, "God gave to us":—

"It is erected in the best style of Chinese architecture, and has an extremely picturesque and attractive appearance. The front building, standing in its own courtyard, is ascended by broad stone steps, which lead from the covered gateway to a verandah, with massive wooden pillars running along its whole length. A hall divides it into two portions. On the right side and in front is a spacious dispensary, which, thanks to the liberality of the Viceroy, is wanting in nothing, rivalling any English dispensary in the abundance and variety of the drugs, appliances, etc. ; behind this is a roomy drug-store. On the left of the hall is a large waiting-room, with benches for the convenience of the patients, and used on Sundays and other days as a preaching hall. Behind, and to one side, is the Chinese reception-room always to be found in a native building. The rooms are very lofty, without ceilings, leaving exposed the huge painted beams, many times larger than foreigners deem necessary, but the pride of the Chinese builder.

" Running off in two parallel wings at the back are the surgery and wards, the latter able to accommodate thirty-six in-patients. The wards in the right wing, four in number, are small, intended each to receive only three patients ; here we can isolate dangerous cases, and also receive persons, such as officials and others, who require greater privacy. The wards are all furnished with kangs instead of beds, as is the custom in North China. These kangs are built of bricks, with flues running underneath, so that in winter they can be heated ; the bedding is spread upon a mat over the warm bricks."

The opening ceremony is thus described :—

" The various rooms were gaily decorated ; the place of honour was reserved for the Chinese Dragon, but a large number of other national flags were also used in draping the walls and ceilings.

" The waiting-room, where the ceremony was to take place, was arranged as a Chinese grand reception-room, the furniture being borrowed from the yamens for the occasion, and the floors covered with camels' hair carpets

" Amongst the Chinese guests were the three Taotais, the Prefect of the city, and numerous civil and military mandarins. The English, German, Russian, and American Consuls were also present.

" Upon the arrival of the Viceroy an illuminated address in Chinese was presented to him. His Excellency, in a few words, expressed his thanks, adding that he was unworthy of so much praise.

" Speeches in Chinese were then delivered by the British and Russian Consuls, and then Mr. Taotai Mah, the Chief Secretary, replied for the Viceroy in French. After the speech-making was concluded, the native assistants were introduced to the Viceroy, who, after formally opening the building, commenced a careful inspection. He examined many varieties of drugs, inquiring into their properties, and wished to know if we had any remedies in common with the Chinese. He asked also if most of our medicinal agents came from the organic or inorganic kingdoms ; about the cost of foreign drugs, and other queries too numerous to mention. But in the surgery the greatest amount of interest was excited. The walls were hung with anatomical and physiological charts ; on the operating-table and shelves were spread the valuable collection of surgical instruments belonging to the hospital, with models of the human body and heart, lent by the Tien-tsin civil doctors. Everything in this department was new, even to such officials as the Viceroy and Superintendent of Arsenals, to whom the latest inventions in electricity and mechanics are

immediately sent.   Although there is no railway in
China, the Viceroy has intelligently studied the steam-
engine from models, and is probably better acquainted
with its working than many well-informed foreigners.

" Questions without number as to the uses, action,
etc., of various instruments were put, and required all
one's readiness of mind to give answers that would be
easily comprehended.   The size of the human brain
in relation to the body, as shown in the wax model,
drew special attention.   After the wards had been
examined, the guests sat down to partake of refreshments ; and it was evident, as each took his departure,
that the Chinese officials went away highly delighted
with their visit.

"On the Sunday following the opening of the
hospital a thanksgiving meeting was held in the
hospital, attended by members of all the churches
in Tien-tsin.

" A number of missionary friends spoke in words of
praise and thanksgiving for what God had manifestly
wrought.   He, of a truth, had heard and answered
prayer, and when the door seemed well-nigh closed,
had opened wide its portals.   Much prayer was
offered up, that as God had already given so many
temporal blessings, and drawn the people so near us,
He would, in the days. that are to come, pour down
richly of those spiritual blessings for which our hearts
are longing."

It was indeed evident to all that the prayers of
those early months had been answered in a most

remarkable manner, for even in the minor needs of the work there were so many of what the world calls coincidences, but Christians the hand of God. Well indeed might the Doctor say, in speaking of these experiences : " I do indeed believe in prayer. I am forced to believe in it, and to say, from practical experience, I am sure that God does hear and answer prayer."

CHAPTER X.

EVANGELISTIC LABOURS.

CHAPTER X

EVANGELISTIC LABOURS.

WE have seen that in less than two years after Dr. Mackenzie's arrival in Tien-tsin he found himself in possession of exceptional advantages for the development of Medical Mission work. It seemed as if the Lord had not only answered His servant's long-continued and earnest prayers, but had given him even more than he had dreamed of. Not only had he a large and well-appointed hospital within the Mission compound, the current expenses of which were all defrayed by the Viceroy ; he had also, in the heart of Tien-tsin city, close to the Viceroy's yamen, a dispensary for out-patients.

But Dr. Mackenzie could never have been contented with these great advantages if he had not had full scope for his work as an evangelist.

" Let us not be satisfied," he wrote in after years, " with mere crowds flocking to us for medical treatment. We have a higher vocation to fulfil. Let us wait expectingly for the touch of faith, and with the Master may this alone satisfy our hearts.

" Our waiting-rooms may be full of patients, and all

14

our beds be occupied, and yet these men and women will pass from under our care pretty much as they came to us, so far as higher things are concerned, unless we directly bestir ourselves for their spiritual good. They seek us, it is true, but for their bodies only ; if we would win their souls, we must seek them. The command to us, as to all the disciples, is ' Go ye,' ' Compel them to come in.' Deliver us from thinking that we are obeying this command when we employ an evangelist, and say to him, ' You go and preach to the patients, while I attend to their bodies.' This is not being a Medical Missionary."

" After all," he writes to a medical friend in China, " our great work lies in bringing home the love of God to our patients. What a glorious thing it is to be engaged in such a service ! Spiritual results can never die, but must go on to eternity."

And in these the early days of the great prosperity which had come to him in so wonderful a way, Mackenzie's one thought seemed to be how he might use every advantage for the glory of his Lord and Master.

" While I am so frequently having conversations with the Viceroy and Lady Li, I need to let them see," he writes, " what true Christianity is like. May God help me, by my conduct and actions, to exemplify the teachings of Jesus. ' Whether believers in Jesus Christ or not,' remarked the Viceroy on one occasion, ' we are all of one mind in wishing to aid in the healing of the sick.' "

This was true ; but the bringing of sin-sick souls for healing to the Great Physician was to Dr. Mackenzie the great end of all his work. A letter which he received about this time from his aged father, and preserved with much care, shows how the home influences which had surrounded his earliest days were of a nature to develop such a spirit of loving consecration.

" May these bodily cures, which you are instrumental and privileged in accomplishing, shadow forth the still greater cure of the diseases of sin which the Great Physician alone can effect. You have indeed great cause for thankfulness in the way in which the Lord hath led you. What an argument for trusting in Him more fully !

" It is very gratifying to hear that you never enjoyed better health ; still you must not overwork yourself, but husband your strength. Your dear mother is sending out to Millie a very precious book called ' John Whom Jesus Loved.' Spurgeon writes very highly of it, as one of those books which a dozen readings will only make more interesting. ' The Lord reigneth.' The whole succession of events is part of the chain of Divine purposes. What if the occurrences that are taking place now in Tien-tsin be a link in that mighty chain of events that will in due time bring about the salvation of China ! "

And God did not disappoint His servant's faith ; He allowed him to see even here great spiritual blessing as the result of his labours.

" One of the first patients in the new hospital," the Doctor writes, "was baptized last week. He was a sinner indeed, with whom no Pharisee would associate ; but ' they that are whole need not a physician.' This man realized his spiritual sickness, and with joy received salvation. He was a subordinate in the Prefect's yamen, named Chow, and got his living by demanding blackmail from the keepers of houses of ill fame. These houses exist against the law, but as they bribe the underlings of the yamens their existence is winked at.

" This man was a general bully and rascal. He came to the hospital to undergo an operation for the cure of caries of the ribs. Having no help at hand, I operated without chloroform, and was struck with the unusual fortitude of the man in bearing pain. He saw the necessity for the operation, and submitted without the slightest flinching. He had a good deal of character, and during his stay of over two months in the hospital he became acquainted with the doctrines of salvation. Side by side with his physical improvement there was undoubtedly a moral change going on within him, visible in the calm, straightforward look of his face. When he went out he had come to the conclusion that he could not return to his old post, although it was still kept open for him, and was a money-making office. Then he tried hard to get other employment, but having learnt no trade this was not an easy matter. Moreover, he had money out at usury, and he found, because he no longer bullied and browbeat, the people refused to pay him either principal or interest. But he still held out, attending the service regularly, and never asking our help. Finally he has got employment which will take him away from Tien-tsin, and so, at his earnest request, he was baptized. I believe he is genuinely sincere, for he has lost much and gained nothing, from a worldly point of view."

Writing for friends at home, the Doctor gives them the following graphic account of his daily work :—

" Let me take you in thought to our Chinese hospital. Ascending a broad flight of stone steps to the verandah, we pass into a lofty hall and enter the waiting-room. Forms are ranged down the whole length of it and at both sides. Texts of Scripture in Chinese decorate the walls, while at one end of the room stands a chair and table.

" The hour is nine o'clock, and the gong is sounding for morning prayers. Already groups of men are collected from the city and villages around, some having their bedding by their side done up in bundles. *There* is a man nearly blind ; his little son has led him here this morning ; *here* sits a lame man, with his crutches in his hand. That pale, hollow-cheeked, feeble man has probably dysentery or phthisis. The sallow, emaciated opium smoker is also there, and one who is suffering from a horrible tumour has come up for operation. As the gong beats the in-patients who are sufficiently convalescent come trooping in ; a strange spectacle indeed, with their bandages and dressings on. Here come the assistants, and now we all take our seats.

"A hymn is given out—perhaps it is one from Sankey's collection, then a portion of Scripture is read, verse about. The subject is probably a Gospel one, very likely a case of healing. It is explained, and lessons are drawn from it ; the patients, who continue to drop in, are generally very quiet and attentive. The meeting closes at the end of half an hour with prayer. Then the medical missionary crosses to the dispensary, while the native evangelist continues to talk to the patients as they wait for their turn. And now the work of healing begins ; one by one the patients come into the dispensary. This is a large room, with two sides occupied with shelves and drawers containing our stock-in-trade. In front is a counter, at which the dispensers are at work putting up medicines. At the table sits the writer, taking down the particulars of each case, and making out the tickets. On one side of the room is a row of chairs and small square tables, a table, or tea-poy, being placed between two chairs.

" Here comes a typical case, led by a friend—a man suffering from eye disease. From the ineffectual attempt he makes to see you his sight is evidently very bad. You examine his inflamed eyes, and find that to protect them from the glare and dust he is constantly contracting his eyelids. The inflammation, therefore, spreads to the lids, which become permanently contracted. The rubbing of the turned-in lids

and lashes upon the tender eyeball leads from bad
to worse, until, from neglect and ignorance, fatal
blindness often results.

" Happily, the case this morning is not of long
standing ; the patient is told that he must become an
in-patient, undergo a slight operation, and there is
every prospect of his sight being greatly improved,
and the probability of a complete cure.

" If the patient is a stranger, at the word operation
he will probably start back in dismay, exclaiming,
'Cut! No, never!' You quietly call to one of the
assistants to lead the patient, with his friend, to one
of the wards to rest awhile. There is sure to be a
similar case under treatment, and the testimony of
one of the man's own countrymen is of more weight
with him than any amount of arguing on our part.
By the time we are ready to operate he has probably made his appearance again, and is smilingly
consenting.

" But we must hurry on, or our morning's work
will not be finished. One by one the patients
follow each other ; the serious cases are urged to
remain, or are told frankly that we can do nothing
for them. The rest have wounds dressed, bandages
or splints applied, and medicines given to them.

" Here comes a man who rushes forward in eager
salutation, dragging behind him a companion ; he
introduces himself as a former patient, and the friend
who accompanies him is willing to submit to any treatment we may propose without demur, his fears having

been entirely removed by his comrade's persuasions.
Here, carried in truly Oriental fashion upon his bed,
or in a basket, is a case of severe palsy, for which we
can do nothing but speak some kind word. Or it
may be a casualty—an accident case from one of
the arsenals or factories. But we have not finished.
Here comes an official's servant with a large red piece
of paper in his hand ; it is his master's visiting card,
and he informs us that the gentleman will soon be
here. Shortly he appears, probably accompanied
by a friend ; he is received at the door, and invited
into the reception room. If he is not very ill, I probably invite him into the dispensary to inspect our
work. In they come, and are seated with some
difficulty, for no one likes to take the upper seat, and
then the inevitable cup of tea is brought. Then their
servants must bring our official friends their pipes
to smoke as they watch us at work. As the patients
pass under review these gentlemen quickly discover
that they have friends suffering from the same com-
plaints. One is certain that a relative has a cough
exactly like that man's, and they will advise these
sick friends immediately to come down for treatment.
When our dispensary work is over, we proceed to
visit the wards. Look at that man sitting on his
brick bed, with his bedding still in a bundle, instead
of being comfortably spread out. He is a new comer,
and has not as yet quite got over his fears. By
to-morrow he will be as jolly as his bodily ailment
allows. By one bedside, as we enter, sits the native

evangelist, with an open Bible upon his knee ; he has been expounding the Scriptures. Portions of Gospels and tracts are scattered about the wards, and as we pass from patient to patient, dressing wounds and attending to the wants of all, we question them upon the books by their side and exhort them to think of the truths of Christianity, and thus have innumerable opportunities for individual dealing.

" I have written of the brick beds, or kangs, and must explain that in the north of China (whatever they do elsewhere) we have in our hospital no spring mattresses, but brick platforms, pierced with a system of flues for heating the beds in the winter.

" I make a rule never to take in hand a case of surgical operation unless there is a very good probability of recovery. But the Chinese stand operations remarkably well, for I have removed a cancerous tumour as large as my hand from a woman of fifty years of age, and the next morning have found her, against all orders, walking about the wards.

" And in these days, though God has not given to His servants miraculous powers of healing, yet so greatly has He enlightened us, that the man fully instructed and doing his work in humble dependence upon Divine help, will achieve such success that in the eyes of the Chinese it appears to be well nigh miraculous."

On Christmas Day, 1880, the Doctor writes to his brother :—

" The Customs Taotai, for whom I had, during

the year, done some work, such as examine patients
for whom he wanted a certificate and so on, sent
me $100 for my own expenses. This fee will go to
increase my reserve fund."

Dr. Mackenzie's ideas about this "reserve fund" are
thus described in a paper he drew up to interest the
Chinese in the new hospital.

"As the object of this free hospital is to aid the
poor, the rich are invited to subscribe, and to some
medicines are sold, the money being placed on
deposit as a reserve fund. It is our wish that this
fund increase so that the hospital may be carried on
as a permanent establishment; and if this is so, there
are emergencies apt to arise, such as buildings requiring repairs, accidents by fire, etc., which would need
to be provided against."

To this account all savings from the allowance of
the Viceroy were placed; also all sums received as
gifts by the Doctor from grateful patients, fees that
came to him from consultations with other physicians
and the like, and it was nursed by careful investments
and economies.

The advisability, or otherwise, of making a charge
for attending patients coming to the Medical Mission
hospitals is a question that has frequently been discussed by missionary physicians. Dr. Mackenzie
gives his own views upon the subject in a letter to
Dr. Dugald Christie of Moukden.

"My own opinion," he says, "is certainly against
making charges for attendance or rooms in hospitals. I

think it tends to hinder freedom in Christian work, and
to give people the idea of the Medical Mission being a
' mai mai ' affair, out of which the foreigner is making
money, and this even though the charge be a small
one. Whereas, on the other hand, I rarely find any
difficulty in showing a well-to-do patient his duty in
subscribing to the hospital. They thoroughly understand a subscription list made in Chinese fashion,
setting forth in the preface the desired object ; and
this I either place in the hands of a patient, or send
it to him at his home. There are blank spaces for
the names of subscribers. I think I once, a long time
ago, put up a notice in each ward, but it did not
work. An individual appeal has to be made, and
sometimes his duty in the matter very clearly pointed
out to a patient."

During the year 1880 there are several references
in Dr. Mackenzie's home letters to the failure of his
wife's health. "This climate seems to agree very
badly with her," he says. "She has never been so
robust as she was in England since coming north."
During the winter no improvement was apparent in
Mrs. Mackenzie's condition, and in February 1881
he wrote to the Foreign Secretary of the London
Missionary Society as follows :—

"It is my very painful duty to inform the Directors
that my wife's health, after long being in a precarious
condition, has at last so broken down that her medical
attendants have ordered her to leave the country at
once, and to return to her native land."

The Doctor accompanied his wife and child to
Shanghai, and saw them on board the *Agamemnon*, in
company with their old Hankow friends Mr. and Mrs.
Taylor, and then returned to his work in Tien-tsin.
This parting was naturally an extremely trying one,
but the feeling of loneliness was, however, kept in
check by constant occupation. About this time he
writes :—

" We have accommodation for thirty-five in-patients,
and we are nearly full. This means a great deal
more than the mere numbers imply. The hospital
cannot be made an asylum for the chronic sick ; we
could fill it over and over again in this way. But
I only admit cases that can be, in all probability,
cured or considerably relieved, and these chiefly surgical cases requiring operations. For such there is
no help in China, excepting in Western surgery, and
I am aiming at making this a resort for all requiring
surgical operations.

" In Tien-tsin there are unusual facilities for help
during the winter. Sometimes gunboats of four
nationalities are in the river, each with its surgeon
on board, and they make our hospital a resort for
clinical and surgical work. Hardly a day passes but
some surgical operations are performed. It is in the
rapid recoveries and successful treatment of hopeless
surgical maladies that the Chinese see the triumph
of Western healing art. It is a glorious thing to see
our wards full of grave cases so generally doing
well. For considering the large number of major

operations, the deaths have been ludicrously small as compared with the tables of mortality from the London hospitals.

" One reason is that the home-surgeon operates if there is only the ghost of a chance ; whereas I reject all hopeless cases, for we have an impression to make, and can't afford to be reckless. But probably a more important reason is, that the nourishing yet simple diet of the Chinese enables them more effectually than an European to resist the shock of an operation.

" Millie talks of my coming home ; but I feel more and more convinced that I am in my right place, and would not change my position very readily. By-and-bye, however, if the work still grows, the London Missionary Society will have to send out another man to help me. There is something being done to break down the prejudices of the influential classes. I will give you an instance that has just happened. Last year I was attending the city Taotai for a bad attack of asthma ; the Viceroy had told him to send for me. While at his house one day he asked me to give his wife some medicine, as she was not well. She then made her appearance for the first time, but she was so timid and nervous that after just feeling her pulse she vanished like a scared rabbit, evidently thinking that I was a dreadfully strange creature, to whom it would be safe to give a wide berth. I suppose she had heard a lot of stories about foreign devils, as we are often called among themselves. At any rate, I could only make out that she had not much the matter with her ; but I

sent her some sugar-coated tonic pills. The next
time I was in the yamen I asked after Mrs. S——.
'Oh, she was no better!' 'Had she taken the pills?'
'Yes, but not all, as they tasted so nastily.'

"Well, I couldn't stand that, as I knew they were
tasteless pills, so I asked to see the box, and, behold,
not one had been taken. She had been afraid to
take them, but the people about couldn't in politeness
say so. Hence I make a rule never to go out to any
but very serious cases. Well, this month the official
had a return of his asthma, and getting no relief sent
for me, and I found him in a terrible condition;
fortunately I could relieve him. Some days later his
wife had a bad attack of quinsey, and finding no
native remedy help her, I was again consulted. This
time she was too ill to run away, and thankfully
attended to my instruction. I saw her frequently, and
she daily improved. She now found that I was not
such an ogre after all. When I saw her the last time,
two days ago, she was quite well, and although her
husband was out she invited me in, showing how
entirely her dread was gone. She asked me a lot
of questions about railways and telegraphs,—how
quickly people could travel by railroad? when the
telegraph was finished, how long would it take to
send a message to her friends in Shanghai and
get an answer back? At last she asked me very
innocently, 'Is it true that you foreign doctors take
people's eyes out and put them back again?' And
then answering herself, said, 'It is not true, is it?'

This lady, between twenty and thirty years of age, is the handsomest woman I have ever seen in China, and when her fear had gone was a perfect lady, and very intelligent.

"Now this lady will in future put all her friends right about that strange creature, the foreign devil. Probably none but medical missionaries, and those only who have gained the confidence of this class, can influence for good in such quarters.

"Now as old patients are leaving, they send up others from the country, or from other towns. One man named Li, who nine months ago entered the hospital nearly blind, and left it with sight restored, arrived yesterday from his home, about forty li away, bringing with him a man who had crushed his hand between two junks. One half of the hand had to be amputated.

"But to return to our friend Li. I have been thinking, during the past week, of engaging an evangelist to seek out the homes of old patients in the country, and strive to follow up the teachings they have received while in the hospital. The right man, a trusty, reliable Tien-tsin Christian, having been found, I have engaged him, and selected the village of the man Li for his first visit. A letter of introduction was written, and he was about to start, when who should arrive but Li himself, with the accident case. I found him delighted at the idea of the evangelist visiting his home. Said he, 'I have been preaching myself to my neighbours, and calling upon them to

give up idolatry and worship the true God, and believe
in Jesus ; but my knowledge is limited, and I cannot
answer the questions they put to me.'   I asked him
if he prayed to God.   ' No,' he replied, ' I have not
the knowledge ; I can't make a prayer.'   ' Is your
father alive ? ' I asked.   ' No,' was his reply.   ' Well,
supposing he was, would you be able to converse with
him, to tell him your difficulties and to seek his help ? '
' Of course I should ! '   ' Well, then, remember that
God is your heavenly Father ; He does not want you
to " make a prayer."   He wants you to seek His help ;
to reverentially converse with Him.'   ' What ! ' said
he, ' can I go down on my knees and tell God that
I am a sinner, and ask Him to help me ; and can I
ask Him to supply my needs ? '   ' Yes,' said I, ' pleading the name and merit of Christ, you can pray to
God for what you want.'   ' Oh, then I understand,'
he replied.   ' I can pray now ! '

   "To-day, in company with the evangelist, Li left
Tien-tsin for home, taking tracts and Scriptures with
them ; I trust that the Lord will greatly bless this
effort.

   "A man named Ku, at present in hospital, has
applied for baptism, and he appears very sincere, and
a humble believer.   Twenty years ago he heard the
gospel in a chapel, and was greatly disturbed there-
with ; but when the massacre took place he ran away
to Pao-ting-fu, for fear he should get into trouble
from being interested in the gospel.   A month ago
he consulted me at the temple dispensary for a

surgical affection. I sent him into the hospital for operation, and he has there learned, I trust, the truth as it is in Jesus, and believed. Many others amongst the in-patients are now seeking admission to the Church, so that we have much to be thankful for.

" I believe the Viceroy to be thoroughly in earnest for the improvement of his country, but what can one man do against a host, even though the one man has extreme power ? He cannot, at his bidding, change the institutions of his country ; and the whole system of government, from top to bottom, is rotten to the core. Nothing can save China but Christianity—a heart religion in place of a hollow morality ; therefore anything that tends to advance the cause of Christ in this land is of supreme importance. Once let China awake from her lethargy, moved by the Spirit of God, purified and in her right mind, and she will become a mighty power in the world. Her immense population, now kept within bounds by repeated famines, floods, and pestilences, under a new *régime* will grow and spread upon the face of the earth. Her enormous wealth will then be opened up, and the Chinese, naturally patient, hardworking, and astute, must become a mighty power.

" Meanwhile, each has his own work to do, and, I trust, nay, I am quite sure, that here in Tien-tsin we are doing something towards the opening up and broadening out of the nation. I am daily meeting with Chinese who have never known foreigners before, and who will form their impressions, in a large

15

measure, from such meetings. What queer notions
the best educated, according to Chinese ideas, have of
us foreigners! By-and-bye they will get to understand us.

"What a mystery is the Christian Church in the
world! England owes everything that is pure, and
virtuous, and truthful, to Christianity ; and yet, outside
the missionary body in China, the number of foreign
residents who pay much respect to religion is so small
as hardly to compose a party.

"Indeed, it is plain, and nowhere plainer than in
China, that a man cannot keep himself. He must be
obedient to some spiritual rule ; either, in his helplessness, he must flee into the arms of his Saviour for
daily protection and guidance, or he will be led captive
of the devil. There may be a middle state in England,
but there is none such possible here. What a merciful
Providence led me to China as a missionary!"

CHAPTER XI.

CHINESE MEDICAL SCHOOL.

CHAPTER XI.

CHINESE MEDICAL SCHOOL.

DR. MACKENZIE'S hands seemed to be already so filled with all-engrossing labour in his unremitting care for the spiritual as well as the bodily needs of his patients, that to most minds it would have seemed almost an impossibility for him to attempt to carry on any additional form of work. And yet when the call of duty came to him, and he saw an open door leading to a sphere, as yet almost untouched by medical missionary effort, the Doctor gladly pressed forward to undertake the work, even though he knew how much of arduous labour it involved.

In a letter to the Foreign Secretary of the London Missionary Society, Mackenzie thus describes the new branch of service which he had undertaken.

"One interesting feature worthy of special remark has been the establishment of a small medical school during the past year. You will no doubt be aware that the Chinese government, about ten years ago, at the instigation of a few of their enlightened men, opened an educational mission in America. They selected from respectable families, chiefly in Canton and Shanghai, lads from ten to twelve years of age, and, under the supervision of Mr. Yung Wing, placed them in the best schools of America. The senior students had all passed through the elementary schools, and had spent two years in college, when last year the mandate went forth from Peking recalling the whole mission.

"This sudden action was due to certain reports having reached the Peking Foreign Office, to the effect that the students were throwing aside the manners and customs of their forefathers, and, in some cases, it was even feared were adopting not only foreign ideas, but also foreign religions. When I heard of their contemplated return I drew up a memorial, requesting the Viceroy to place eight of these students under my charge for the study of medicine and surgery, with a view to their being utilized eventually as medical officers by the Government.

This proposition was agreed to, and upon the arrival of the students in Tien-tsin eight of them were accordingly handed over to my charge.

" Being wholly under Christian influence, it is our earnest prayer that they may leave our hands enlightened spiritually as well as medically.

" Of course the establishment of this school, although so small at present, necessarily greatly increases my work ; but I felt that the opportunity was one that should not be missed   We want to reach the educated classes of this land, and it is one way of doing so."

Speaking of the desirability of commencing this medical school, the Doctor says :—

"Of course it is beyond question that until the Chinese Government is prepared to establish a fully equipped medical college, with a complete staff of teachers, it would be better policy for them to send a batch of students to some European or American medical school for training. But it was evident that even our enlightened Viceroy was not prepared for such a step as this, and we therefore proposed a scheme likely to be sanctioned, rather than one that would inevitably have been shelved."

A few days after, the Doctor writes :—

"The scheme has been accepted. So the first Government medical school in China will now be started, in a small way at first ; yet it is a beginning. I shall have my hands full, however ; it is thought enough at home to lecture upon one subject, such as physiology ; but I shall have to teach subjects all round. Yet there was no withdrawing from the responsibility, unless I was prepared to see things going on as they are, when I had it in my power to start a change in the right direction. In fact, I rather enjoy the idea of being compelled to tackle the subject, for I know that in teaching others I shall be best taught myself ; probably by next year the way will be open to enlarge the scheme, and get help from home ; but time will tell."

Writing some years after, Dr. Mackenzie thus describes this medical school, and the progress it had made :—

"The school was inaugurated on December 15th,

1881, under the Chinese title of the ' I-hsuch-kwan.'
The students, having been brought up in cultured
American homes and schools, had all received a good
English education, and were trained to study.

" The teaching is conducted much as general school
work is done at home.   Each pupil, having his own
class books, prepares a given amount, and is examined
in it daily, while his instructor explains and illustrates
the text.   For the first set of students the teaching
was mainly in my hands, though for a period of eight
months Dr. Atterbury of Peking had the entire charge
and instruction of them, he having in the most generous
way given his services in a time of great need.   And
well nigh without an exception, most of the medical
officers belonging to the American and English navies
resident in the port of Tien-tsin during the winter
months, have rendered valuable help in the training
of the pupils.   Examinations have been held three
times a year, in the presence of H. E. the Customs
Taotai, and an English-speaking official appointed by
the Viceroy, and conducted by independent medical
men, both orally and by written papers.   At the
examinations, especially the important ones consti-
tuting the ' Primary ' and ' Pass,' the former held at
the completion of eighteen months of almost continuous study, and the latter at the end of the curri-
culum, the school has been indebted to Drs. Frazer
and Irwin, whose ready sympathy and kindly help on
so many occasions I cannot too gratefully acknowledge.   These gentlemen, together with the naval

officers above mentioned, and any medical missionaries staying for the time being in Tien-tsin, have constituted the Board of Examiners. The certificates given at the primary examination of the first class were signed by, Andrew Irwin, Customs Medical Officer, Tien-tsin ; Arthur G. Cabell, P.A., Surgeon U. S. Navy ; Thomas Edward H. Williams, Surgeon Royal Navy, as examiners ; and by John Kenneth Mackenzie, Medical Officer, Viceroy's Hospital, as tutor."

" I do not value this branch of work so much from the medical side," the Doctor writes to a friend in England. " If it merely meant training surgeons for the Chinese Government I would give it up. I value it as a rare means of influencing these educated young men from a Christian standpoint. My hands are left perfectly free by the Viceroy, and the young men are entirely under my charge."

Later on he writes :—

" The work is very interesting and instructive to myself. We have a Debating Society every Saturday evening, when we take up a variety of topics for discussion. ' Which was the greater man, Cæsar or Napoleon ? ' was the subject of one debate. The meeting decided in favour of Cæsar. On another occasion, whether Paul was greater than Moses was discussed, and the larger number of votes was given to Moses. On Sunday a very successful class of students meets in my house to discuss, or rather to search, the Scriptures. They have certainly a clear knowledge of the gospel, and in the case of two at least we feel assured a spiritual change has come about.

"While I enjoy the work among the students, and feel that it is a field we can so seldom enter upon in China, namely, getting into close contact with the highly educated, and thus influencing them, as I trust God is enabling us to do, in some measure, in every case, yet it sorely taxes my time. Anatomy, physiology, medicine, surgery, besides the allied branches, to be all taught by one individual means incessant study for oneself. Of course I am getting repaid again and again in clearer knowledge, and in the rich pleasure which is derived from work of almost any kind if useful."

It will be seen that the life Dr. Mackenzie was living was indeed a busy one. Not only had he the sole care of the hospital, constantly filled with patients, resting upon him, and the after-strain of watching over numberless cases where serious operations had been performed ; he was also, as some one has said, "a whole medical faculty in himself," having the entire care of training the medical students ; and it was also his joy and delight to occupy his spare moments with the evangelistic work which ever lay so near his heart. He was at the same time in robust health, and his heart was gladdened with the news that his wife was restored to health again, and that she, with their little daughter, was hoping to join him in the autumn.

"I was never better than I am at present," he

writes; " I attribute it largely to early rising and taking active exercise on horseback. This is my only re-creation, and I come back feeling fit for any amount of work. One of our prominent medical writers, Lauder Brunton, said lately in the *Practitioner* that ' the best thing for the inside of a man was the outside of a horse,' and there is a lot of sound philosophy in the remark ; I can testify from personal experience."

The Doctor suffered a severe bereavement in the removal by death of his beloved mother towards the end of 1881, and writing to his aged father, who was greatly desiring to see his son once more, in a letter dated August 25th, 1882, he says :—

" This is my birthday, so I must write you a line. I am thirty-two years old to-day, having spent over seven years in China. This is a good slice out of my life, and I heartily wish I could have found it possible, after so long an absence, to visit home and see all your dear faces again. I cannot help thinking of dear mother, for to-morrow was her birthday, and the two days coming so closely together always led me to think especially of her dear face at such a time as this.

" The hospital work goes on as actively as ever, and the little medical school keeps me busy. Truth is being made known to numbers who seek, in the first place, only medical help. Mission work in China is all uphill work ; this one must expect after getting some knowledge of the national character. Yet, nevertheless, genuine and necessary work is being done, and will tell in the long run. The more I know of the Chinese, especially of their educated men, the more I feel that there is a mine of wealth here. The leaven will take long to spread, but it is already at work. The inhabitants of the Pacific Islands are rapidly influenced in comparison with the Chinese, but though the process here will be slower, it will be far mightier in results."

In a later letter to his brother the Doctor says :—

" I have had a visit this morning from a Corean prince and suite. He is now in Tien-tsin arranging the Japan-Corean difficulty, and was sent by the Viceroy to consult me, and also to see the hospital as one of the sights of Tien-tsin. He is a fine gentlemanly man, very sedate and composed. I showed him the house, and Laura Lees and Gertie Stanley played a duet on the piano for him. He looked, too, at some photographs under the microscope, and was greatly surprised to see a little spot develop into fifty persons in full uniform, for one of the photographs was the Duke of Wellington and staff. He also saw models and a human skeleton for the first time."

It was in November of this year that Dr. Mackenzie went down to Shanghai to meet his wife, who had been, with their little daughter, residing in England for more than eighteen months, in the hope that the climate of her native land would restore her to health again. The medical reports had been very favourable, and it was with much satisfaction that Dr. Mackenzie looked forward to having his lonely China home once more gladdened by the presence of wife and child. These bright hopes were, however, doomed to disappointment, and when the Doctor met his beloved wife again, after the long period of separation, he found that during the voyage more serious symptoms had developed themselves, and it seemed very doubtful whether it would be possible for her to remain in China. Some of the medical men in Shanghai thought it likely that after the long voyage the quiet and rest of her own home might prove beneficial to the invalid.

So, as he said himself, "hoping almost against hope," Dr. Mackenzie journeyed northwards with his sick wife and little child. In a very short time, however, it became clear that it was absolutely necessary for Mrs. Mackenzie to return to England, and her state of health was so serious that her husband and all their friends in the mission felt it was his duty to accompany her.

It was with a sad heart that the Doctor made arrangements for leaving, for as short a period as possible, the work he so dearly loved, and the little daughter, who had been taken into the motherly care of Mrs. Lees. The Doctor and his wife sailed for England in the *Glenavon*, which left Shanghai on December 7th, and after a very long voyage arrived in London on February 18th, 1883.

Dr. Mackenzie only remained five months in England, and during a considerable portion of that time was busily engaged in deputation work in various parts of the country. He visited Gloucester,

Cheltenham, Reading, Haverfordwest, Dorking, Hull, Nottingham, and various parts of London.

He occupied the pulpits of the principal Congregational Churches of these places on the Sundays, and greatly interested the people by the story of how God had so wonderfully answered prayer and provided for all the needs of the Tien-tsin Medical Mission. This visit home, though shadowed by the heavy sorrow of his wife's continued illness, was a source of great interest and pleasure to large numbers of Christian people, whose memory of his work and noble character is still vivid and affectionately cherished.

" I wish that my recollection of the details of Dr. Mackenzie's visit were as full and accurate as my impression of his character is clear and strong," writes a friend, whose guest he was during a visit to his city. " His earnestness, sincerity, humility, and loving faith were unmistakable. He did not enjoy the Sunday preaching, which was part of his deputation work here, but he had large and interested congregations. Every one to whom I have spoken seems to remember all the services with interest, and to have been deeply impressed by Dr. Mackenzie's personality. I shall never forget one striking instance of his humility. He was the last speaker at a crowded missionary meeting, which had gone on rather quietly, when he began, and raised the large audience to a perfect glow of enthusiasm. Immediately afterwards he said to me how much he wished that people knew and cared more about the missionary work. I, speaking out of the fulness of my heart, replied, ' They soon would if we had more speeches like that.' He instantly answered, in quite a pained voice, ' Oh, don't say that ; you would not if you knew.' I could not but feel grieved to have wounded him, but it was true. If he was only the instrument, there was such a large measure of the power that cometh from above that none were unmoved. I think the charm of Dr. Mackenzie's life lay partly in its unity. Apparently there were no contending forces. Absolute self-abnegation left room for humility, love, and trust. Medical work was done as carefully as though the issues depended upon that alone ; but the prayer of faith was as earnest as that of any of the so-called ' faith healers.' "

Another lady, a member of Streatham Hill Congregational Church, after writing in similar terms of her impression of Dr. Mackenzie's character, continues : " I remember quite well that the elder boys in my class were so interested, that two of them told me how they should like to go back with him to China to learn surgery and do mission work as well. He had told them of a Chinese young men's class he had in training, to help him in the hospital when they were fit for it."

Before returning to his work in China Dr. Mackenzie, in company with his brother, took a trip on the Continent. They visited Antwerp, Brussels, and Cologne ; gazed upon the beauties of Lakes Lucerne and Zurich, and wandered among the Swiss valleys and glorious mountain peaks. This tour seems to have been a source of great delight and enjoyment to the Doctor. He returned to England by the middle of July, and on the 31st of that month set sail alone for China in the *SS. Glencoe.* Mrs. Mackenzie's state of health seemed to indicate that it would not be possible for her, for a considerable time, if ever, to return to the East. This separation from his wife, and the consequent breaking up of his home, was the sorrow which saddened all Mackenzie's after life. No trial, perhaps, could have been harder to bear to one whose nature was so deeply affectionate, and who felt that God had so clearly called him to carry on the medical work in Tien-tsin, and had blessed that work with such special marks of Divine favour ; yet, as is so often the case, when the heart has learned the blessed secret of casting all earthly sorrows on an unseen yet ever-living Redeemer, the chastisement yielded afterwards the peaceable fruits of righteousness, and did much towards the development and making of his spiritual life, while his personal griefs only made him better able to enter into the sorrows of others.

The voyage seems to have been, on the whole, a favourable one, although intense heat was experienced in the Red Sea, and somewhat rough weather in the Indian Ocean.

" We are a very happy party," he writes to his brother. " I should hardly have thought a sea voyage would have gone so pleasantly. The doctor is a good fellow, and I like him much. I finished the eighth volume of Froude this morning; I have greatly enjoyed it, and have obtained quite a new idea of Henry VIII. and Elizabeth. It is pleasantly written too, and not too dry for reading on ship board."

"You will have heard by telegraph," he writes in the China Sea, " that there has been a frightful earthquake in Java, and over a radius of fifty miles. The shock was felt at Singapore, a distance of six hundred miles. One island, thirteen miles round, with a mountain three thousand feet high, has disappeared. The whole aspect of the coast has been quite altered, and lighthouses have been destroyed, so that captains are notified that navigation will not be safe until the whole district has been again surveyed and fresh charts drawn out.

"An Australian steamer lying next to us in Singapore reported passing through floating corpses in every direction. The shock was accompanied by two enormous tidal waves, the waters rising a height of seventy feet, and carrying everything away before them. One English lady was saved by being lodged in the top of a high cocoanut tree. The number of deaths is estimated at thirty thousand."

On September 12th he continues :—

" Here we are at Hong-Kong, after a very stormy day and night. We were in the wake of a typhoon all day yesterday. They tell us here that a typhoon has lasted three days, but is now over. All the shipping in harbour is made firm with many anchors.

"As we have to stay three days here I thought of spending the time by going up to Canton, but I find by the papers that a riot took place there two days ago, a plot to murder the Europeans having been got up; so I won't go yet."

He decided afterwards to go to Canton, however, in company with Dr. Chalmers, and thus describes the state of matters there :—

"The English settlement was in ruins ; that is, out of thirty handsome buildings fifteen were totally destroyed by fire and others had been looted. The mob had risen and done this damage to property. The cause of the rising was said to be the brutality of some rough Englishman. There is generally some such cause to account for these riots. One Chinaman had been shot by an Englishman, and within a few days another man was pushed or kicked from an English steamer lying at Canton, and falling into the water, was drowned. When this second death occurred the mob saturated the wharf with kerosene oil, and then set fire to it, in the hope of igniting the steamer, but she got away into the stream.

"In a mad rage the crowd broke up a kerosene depôt, and carried off tins of the inflammable oil to the English settlement, and very shortly fifteen houses, with all their contents, had been utterly destroyed. By the time troops had arrived from the camp the mob had entirely disappeared. It is a marvel that no

European lives were lost. The residents, men and women, had to escape as best they could to the steamers. We dined with the Consul, whose house was untouched. The mob came into his grounds, when he immediately lowered his flag, and they, seeing the flag, left his house, evidently fearing to involve the Government too far. The London Mission houses in the settlement were looted, but not fired, and the other missionary houses in the native city were untouched. Dr. Kerr has had a Mission hospital for many years in one part of the city, and there are three Mission houses there. When the news of the rising came the Chinese neighbours collected, and barricaded the streets to keep away the mob if they attempted to attack the property, but they made no attempt to interfere with any of the Mission houses in the city.

" A letter was awaiting me at Hong-Kong from Lees, giving me all news, and saying that Maggie was in the best of health and spirits. He enclosed a letter from the Tien-tsin Taotai, asking me to try and find four English-speaking students to join our medical school, and sending me an introduction to the head of the Hong-Kong Central School, a large Government institution in connection with the colony. The offer was made, and I selected four from eleven applicants. They are to follow me as soon as the permission of the governor has been obtained. Upon my arrival in Hong-Kong I heard a most sad piece of news. Dr. Schofield died of typhus fever very suddenly in Tai-

yuen-fu.   It is one of the most painful pieces of news
I could have heard.   He was such a splendid man,
and so useful in his position there."

Dr. Mackenzie arrived in Tien-tsin on September
25th, and found a letter awaiting him from the
widow of the lamented Dr. Schofield.   In it she says :
" He sent to you, as to all his friends, his loving farewell, and this one verse of a hymn,—

> 'A little while for winning souls to Jesus,
> Ere we behold His beauty face to face ;
> A little while for healing soul diseases,
> By telling others of a Saviour's grace.'"

The little daughter whom Dr. Mackenzie rejoined
in China remained under the kind care of Mrs. Lees,
and was the solace of his rare intervals of leisure, for
the Doctor soon found himself, as formerly, over-
whelmed with work on all sides.

In December 1883, some three months after his
return to Tien-tsin, the Doctor writes to his brother :—

" I am busily occupied with work ; in fact, I have no
spare time to speak of, yet I enjoy it, and though low-
spirited at times, I am very happy.   The Christian
work goes on very, very slowly here in the north, but
our duty is to continue and to persevere in faith."

With relation to the troubles in Tonquin between
the French and Chinese the Doctor writes : --

" The war news continues very threatening, but I
am still doubtful whether anything will come out of it.
We are closed in for the winter from the outer world,

and probably this will be the last letter sent from Taku this year.

"Last week I made a trust deed, with the aid of our Consul, placing seven thousand taels (£2,000) on trust as a reserve fund for our hospital, to be used (the interest only) in the work of Christian Medical Missions. It is bound down by careful stipulation, so that it cannot be used for other objects. Mr. Lees and myself are the first trustees.

"This money, as you know, I had received from the Chinese, and thought it better to arrange it legally, in case of any changes coming about. The deed I have sent to the London Missionary Society for them to keep in charge. No doubt the value of property in Tien-tsin will increase vastly when foreign improvements are fully introduced in this, the port of the capital. So that in making these arrangements I am looking forward to the interest some day being very large, say in fifty years time, for China, I am con· vinced, has a great future before her."

CHAPTER XII.

SIGNS OF PROGRESS.

CHAPTER XII.

SIGNS OF PROGRESS.

IN October of the year 1884 six of the first batch of students in the Tien-tsin medical school passed their final examination, after three years' study, and received diplomas.

The Viceroy obtained for these men the favour of civil instead of military rank, and gave the head student a crystal button, while on the remaining five was conferred slightly lower rank with white buttons. In a land like China this was a matter of considerable importance, since it affected so materially the social position of the recipient.

Writing some time after to a Chinese medical journal, Dr. Mackenzie gives an interesting account of the after-career of these young surgeons, exemplifying the many difficulties which obstruct the path of progress in this land.

" We want no experiments," he writes, " to show us that Chinese youths are capable of acquiring a scientific education ; what we do want is some evidence that the powers that be will appreciate it when obtained.

"The head of the class was permanently appointed to the school and hospital, and renders valuable assistance both in the instruction of students and the treatment of patients. A second was for some time attached to the medical school, but he now holds the position of medical officer to the new military college in Tien-tsin, where he has the oversight of some two hundred students. This is a good appointment, but is unfortunately underpaid. A third was placed at the service of General Chow, who has the command of a body of troops said to number fifteen thousand, encamped some twenty miles from Tien-tsin. Soon after he had joined the general's staff, an interesting though curious and possibly unique experience awaited him. At the central camp, where the general's headquarters were located, there resided a native doctor, who professed to treat upon foreign principles, but his practice fell sadly short of his profession, indeed it was of the most elementary kind, consisting in the administration of a few simple drugs, backed up by much skill in rhetoric. He had the faculty of adapting his medicines to the theoretic notions of his patients, which is in China a great gift.

"The question arose, should the newly-arrived man be retained at headquarters and the old occupant of the post be removed to another camp, or should the new-comer be placed elsewhere? A brilliant idea originated in the mind of the great man. He himself, aided by the other red-buttoned generals under his command, would sit as a sort of court of inquiry and investigate into the respective abilities of each. The order went forth, and on a fixed day, under a canvas pavilion erected for the occasion, the generals and colonels, attended by their respective staffs—and even a colonel requires a staff in China—assembled in full paraphernalia, and seated themselves in order of precedence. The two unfortunate medicos were then called in, and before this august assembly, and in the presence of each other, underwent an examination, the court putting the questions and deciding the verdict. Each candidate for the favour of the court was expected to show all he knew ; but considering that one of the parties was an astute man of the world, of fifty odd summers, equally conversant with Chinese etiquette and with Chinese ideas of anatomy and disease, while the other had not long entered upon man's estate, whose knowledge of human nature was drawn from the standpoint of the American youth of the nineteenth century, while his anatomical and medical learning, though agreeing with that of the Western schools, differed *in toto* from the innate knowledge held by his examiners, the result may readily be imagined. The elder was adjudged the victor, and was retained at his post, while the younger was placed at a small cavalry camp some distance away. The examiners, scarce one of whom could read or write, as became men who have to wield the sword rather than the pen, returned to their quarters, satisfied, no doubt, that they had upheld the dignity of their country. This surgeon is, however, comfortably situated, having better allowances than any of his fellow-students, and complaining chiefly that he has too little to do.

"A fourth entered the navy, and is now surgeon on board one of the cruisers ; but he is greatly dissatisfied with his position. He sees the executive officers and engineers, many of them his old comrades in America, promoted in rank and pay, while he remains stationary, with no prospect of his position improving unless a war breaks out.

"When they leave the hospital each successful student is provided with a good set of surgical instruments and a supply of drugs sufficient to start him with.

"The fifth was appointed to a camp in the northern part of the coast. While his drugs lasted he was very popular. He opened a dispensary, and had numerous patients daily, but when in course of time his stock began to diminish, and he applied to the general under whose charge he was placed for a fresh supply, his difficulties commenced. He was urged to write and get more drugs from his old hospital, and every imaginable excuse was invented, but no money was forthcoming for supplies. Then it was alleged that Chinese doctoring was cheaper than foreign, and it was discovered that a relative of the general's was a native doctor in the camp. By-and-bye his original stock gave out, and his dispensary had to be closed. For several months he was idle. He appealed to me for help, and I did what I could for him. Finally his relations with his commanding officer became so strained, that he begged to be removed to another position, and his request being granted, he was transferred to the navy. Here again he found that things did not run smoothly, so some months ago he sought and obtained leave of absence, from which he has not returned. I heard later that he had received, through the help of friends, the position of interpreter to one of China's consulates abroad.

" The sixth was likewise attached to the navy, but after serving for some eighteen months, he too retired upon plea of leave of absence, and obtained a more congenial situation ashore

" Thus two out of the six who completed their course have, for the time being, abandoned their profession ; yet I believe that in both cases they would prefer, under more favourable circumstances, to continue the practice of medicine. But they have to contend against many real difficulties. In the first place, the pay is too meagre ; it averages about tls. 30 a month ; and such men find they can command larger salaries in comfortable business positions on land. Then, again, trouble commences whenever they have to draw allowances for drugs, etc., from their commanding officer. A Chinese doctor's services can be obtained for about tls. 7 a month, while the patient pays for his own medicines, thus relieving the mandarin of the obligation of disbursing these payments.

" In the navy especially the *raison d'être* of the surgeon's presence is hardly yet recognized. The crew of a ship of war is presumably composed of able-bodied men, so that in times of peace the post of surgeon on board, even in Western navies, is not a very arduous one ; but he is there in readiness for the exigencies of war. Now the average Chinese captain fails to grasp this idea. He sees the surgeon drawing his pay and having perhaps an easy time of it, and he cannot possibly see the necessity of his presence. It is too far for him to look ahead and contemplate the value of the help to be given by trained men in times of warfare. Viewing the medical man, therefore, somewhat in the light of a useless loafer, is it to be wondered at that the latter's position on board becomes far from enviable, and ceasing to esteem it an honour to serve king and country, he takes the first favourable opportunity of retiring from the Service ?

" Things will not work smoothly and satisfaction prevail until the Government establishes a distinct department for its medical officers, allowing them to draw supplies from central depôts, and arranging a fair scale of salaries and promotion, which will give stability to the service and a career to the men."

It was at the end of 1884 that, under the stress of difficulties with France and the possibility of war being pushed forward into North China, the Viceroy determined upon the addition of a larger number of students to the school ; twelve young men were obtained from the Hong-Kong Central School, and commenced their studies in Tien-tsin.

His Excellency was extremely anxious that the young men's residence should be in close proximity to the Doctor, so that he might be able to have constant oversight of them. He accordingly made a grant for transforming the hospital wards into separate sleeping and class-rooms for students, and at the same time built, on the opposite side of the road, a fine new hospital, to accommodate fifty-five in-patients, and handed it over to Dr. Mackenzie.

" The new building is a great improvement upon the old one," he writes, " for during the last four years I have gained experience of the sort of thing we want in Tien-tsin, and so was able to work in improvements."

From a letter written to the Board at home at this period we find that the Doctor's mind had been much exercised as to the advisability or otherwise of this step.

" I have been a good deal concerned of late," he writes, " as to my duty in regard to medical teaching. The Directors are probably aware that these students are intended for Government service. Now I would not wish to spend my time in merely raising up a band of surgeons for the Chinese Government, and since this autumn the first batch of students have completed their three years' term, I thought it would be a good opportunity for gradually drawing out of the work, and so I should be enabled to devote more time to direct evangelistic labour. On the other hand, most of my friends have strongly urged me to continue the school, considering it to be one of the best forms of missionary effort. I have been led, finally, to see that this is my line of duty, at any rate for the present. Some of the reasons that have influenced me are as follows :—

"(1) The slow progress and very limited success, at present, of direct evangelistic work in North China.

"(2) The extreme difficulty of reaching, through preaching, the educated youth of China.

"(3) That in the Providence of God these educated young men have been placed under my charge without any restrictions or limitations, and so can be instructed in and influenced by Christian truth. Of the present class four are Christians, while others are well inclined, and attend our Bible class with regularity. The Christians hold a daily morning prayer-meeting together.

" Our senior student, Mr. Lin, has already received his appointment as one of the assistant-masters.

" One other reason for the continuance of this class. I look upon the country stations as the most hopeful part of the North China Mission. The simple-minded peasants of the interior are drawn to accept the gospel far more readily than their acuter yet worldly-minded fellow-countrymen in the large towns. Now I am hoping, that with two well-qualified, English-taught Chinese doctors attached to the hospital, I shall be able to get away once or twice each year for a month's visit to our country stations, and so help along my brethren in this most hopeful field. Without the help of my old pupils I should be, as before, tied to the hospital. Every expense in connection with the teaching department is borne by the Chinese officials in the most liberal manner, and their interest in our hospital continues to be kept up. I feel especially thankful for the increased measure of success which has followed the evangelistic work in connection with our in-patients during the past year. As the object of our united effort is the winning of the Chinese for Christ, it is not desirable, I think, to attempt too closely to count up how many converts come from one branch and how many from another branch of our Mission. You will be glad to know, however, that Mr. Lees has already, during the five months of the present year, baptized more converts than during the whole of last year.

" Referring again to the Hospital Reserve Fund, I would first mention that since the deed was drawn up I have been able to add tls. 1,000. This makes the Fund now amount in all to tls. 8,000. I don't think it would be a desirable thing to accumulate too large an endowment for the hospital ; indeed, I have long hoped that the interest might soon be applied to the payment of my salary as medical missionary in charge of the hospital, and so relieve the Directors to this extent."

He goes on, however, to explain that another

proposal has been under consideration by his colleagues, *i.e.*, that in the coming spring the Directors should appoint a medical missionary for the country stations, to work in connection with the Tien-tsin committee. This work of training successive classes of young men in medicine and surgery, which, it has been seen, was not undertaken without much heart-searching and prayer for guidance, was not without signs of blessing from the Master's hand.

"We have several bright Christians in the school," writes the Doctor towards the end of 1885. "Two of those who came here as heathen have been baptized by Mr. Lees in the native church. Three others are the sons of Christian parents, and were baptized as infants, two of them in connection with the Hong-Kong Church." Of another he writes : "His spiritual life has grown very much since coming here, and he is now an aggressive Christian." Somewhat later he writes : "Another of our students has been added to the praying band. It is truly a precious privilege to watch souls expand and grow. Our Christian medical students are in the hot glow of their first love ; the study of the Word of God is their joy. Sunday evening after service we are together going through Hebrews, comparing scripture with scripture ; it is very enjoyable. There is much cause for rejoicing as one looks back upon the year that is past."

In recognition of the abundant services so freely rendered to the students of the medical school, His Excellency the Viceroy having mentioned the matter

in a memorial to the throne, the Emperor was pleased
to confer upon Dr. Mackenzie an Imperial decoration,
" The Star of the Order of the Double Dragon," with
a Chinese commission. Writing at this time to his
brother, the Doctor says :—

" It is a special order, which was instituted some
years ago for bestowal on foreigners. It is called a
star, though it is more square than round. It is made
of gold, with a precious stone set in the centre ; this
stone is blue, and corresponds with the blue button
worn by mandarins, and surrounding the stone are two
dragons.

" There are six characters on the front of it, two
meaning ' Double Dragon,' two meaning ' Precious
Star,' and two more ' Presented by the Emperor.' It
was accompanied by an embroidered ribbon, to be
worn with it, and the whole was encased in an ebony
cabinet, with a despatch to explain the reason of the
gift. It is kindly meant and a gracious gift, and as
such I value it. In Chinese official society, too, it
gives me a certain rank, which is not to be despised
by one living and working here."

The hospital's power as a gospel agency was growing year by year. Dr. Mackenzie's bright example
acted as an inspiration to the hospital workers,
binding them together as fellow-labourers in the
Lord, their one desire being to lead to Christ those
who came within its walls.

" One of our helpers is, I think, a striking instance
of a man born again—born from above," writes the

Doctor. " His name is Yang Ming, and he comes from the province of Shan-tung. He came to us some two years ago suffering from an enormous tumour of the scalp—elephantiasis arabum. It had existed since childhood. He could do no work, could get very little sleep, and latterly suffered much pain from pressure of the tumour on the upper part of the spine. He had received no sort of education, and, with his peculiar deformity, had a very repulsive and animal-like appearance. Speaking his local patois, it was difficult to understand him, and he seemed scarcely capable of taking in an idea. Well, the tumour was removed in three operations, at intervals of a month or so, it being unwise, from the large base of the tumour and the great loss of blood, to remove it at one sitting. He necessarily remained in the wards for a long time, and when he was quite well we offered to engage him as a helper in the wards. He had undergone not only a physical but an intellectual and spiritual change of a very marked kind. His soul, of the possession of which he was not aware when he came, is clearly alive in him, and his mind, so long torpid, has awoke to consciousness. It is now a pleasure to hear him speak about spiritual things, and to see how he has been taught of the Spirit of God. Of course he makes many mistakes, and often gets out of his depth, but what young believer does not ?

" Another striking answer to prayer was when, in 1884, God sent me Chang-Yung-mao as a dispenser. I had been praying for a dispenser, but especially one sent of God, who should do work for Him. This young Christian was in Mr. Lees' theological training school, and was led to volunteer for dispensary work. Since joining us he has thrown new life into the evangelistic work among the in-patients, stimulating the paid evangelist, who gives his whole time to this department, by his zeal and faith. Though his work is that of a dispenser, he devotes his spare time to Christian work. It is telling grandly, and God is blessing him richly in his own soul. I thank God there is an aroma of prayer about the place.

"We now make definite prayer that the Lord will send to the hospital, for the patients come from several hundred miles around, those whom He is calling from among this people. A Christian brother is engaged in visiting the homes of those who have shown an interest in Christian truth while in the hospital."

This man, by name Chang-Yung-tsing, is thus referred to in the report of another member of the Mission, written at the same time:—

"A large number of those baptized in recent years have been men who came from a distance to the hospital as in-patients, and who, on returning home, were lost sight of. To remedy this state of things, Dr. Mackenzie personally employed a Christian for a few months in visiting these scattered disciples. Then the Church took the matter up, and by an additional number of monthly contributions, and being relieved of the payment of the chapel-keeper, they undertook to support a travelling preacher.

Their choice fell unanimously upon a man who, many
years ago, was an agent of the Society, but who soon
gave it up, choosing, like Paul, to be above all suspicion as to his motives for preaching the gospel.
Since then he has been a voluntary labourer, going
up and down the country proclaiming everywhere the
forgiveness of sins in the name of Jesus, and has been
the means of planting the gospel in several villages.
A man with the use only of one eye, and a most
unprepossessing appearance, uncouth in dress and
speech, and naturally of a most stubborn temper, he
is possessed of a warm heart, full of love to Christ and
the souls of men, and though belonging to the illiterate
class, has by diligence acquired an extensive acquaintance with the Word of God, which is more to him
than his daily food.　The only fear which was enter-
tained in selecting Chang-Yung-tsing was, that in
his love of freedom he might refuse even to become
the servant of the native Church.　However, a friendly
invitation being addressed to him, he came to Tien-tsin
and accepted the call."

From the earliest days of his life in China Dr.
Mackenzie's aim had ever been to give prominence to
the evangelistic side of hospital work, and not to be
satisfied with the mere healing of the bodily diseases
of his patients.　And as the years passed on it was
evident to all that this thought was becoming more
and more the ruling principle of all his work, and this
was especially noticeable during the last two or three
years of his life.

At about this time he gives the following account of the evangelistic work carried on in the wards :—

" Let me tell you something of the direct missionary work of the hospital. We have a Scripture reader, paid out of the hospital funds, who devotes his whole time to Christian teaching among the patients. His great work is that of teaching the catechism, for our patients, when they enter, with very rare exceptions, have not even heard the name of God. Many of them cannot read, and he, therefore, instructs those who are willing to learn, so that when they leave quite a large number who did not know a character of the written language can read in the catechism the fundamental truths of the gospel. I conduct every morning, excepting on Sundays, a Bible class among the in-patients and employées of the hospital and dispensary. It lasts for from three-quarters of an hour to an hour, commencing in winter at 8.15, and finishing at 9 or 9.15."

Writing of this meeting some time afterwards, the Doctor says :—

" We make it as conversational as possible, by asking and soliciting questions, and inducing as many as are willing to take part. On Tuesday evenings we hold a class, in which we try to gather up the work of the week, ' drawing up the gospel net,' as it has been well termed, and on Friday evenings there is a special meeting for the helpers and other Christians for prayer and the study of the Scriptures, the medical missionary being the leader at these various classes."

In April 1885 Dr. Mackenzie made the acquaintance of Messrs. Stanley Smith, Hoste, and Cassels,
who stayed at Tien-tsin for several days, *en route* to
Peking.

"We have had delightful meetings for the past
five days," he writes in his diary. "God has been
present, and a great blessing has come down upon
the missionary brethren. It has been a time of
great joy to me, and souls have been saved. Several
of my students in the medical school have been
impressed, and some have confessed Christ."

In relation to this visit, in a letter to a friend in
England the Doctor says :—

"Let me tell you an incident of Stanley Smith's
visit. One day they were going through the hospital,
when I pointed out a case I could do nothing for.
Devil possession, I believe, is the best term for it.
The man had recently arrived, with some friends,
from his home a long way off. Stanley Smith suggested prayer ; so we all prayed for him, and in
God's love I believe he was restored to his right mind.
Next morning he came in to our Bible-reading, and
sat calmly through the meeting. His friends considered he had been cured in answer to prayer, and
they earnestly studied the Word for some days before
returning home."

At another time Dr. Mackenzie wrote :—

"We hear much of faith healing in these days, and
in my opinion the Medical Missionary should be a
faith healer. He should give all the attention possible

to his cases, use every means he can think of, every agency or drug that he knows of ; but he should also do so in humble dependence upon God for His blessing. Just as the ordained preacher should never stand up to deliver his message without looking to the Master for the spiritual influence, so the medical missionary should never perform an operation without seeking the help of Him who is mighty to save. Then, as the one missionary is a faith worker, the other is a faith healer. You have a broken limb brought into your hospital. What is your duty? Why, to use all your skill, your utmost knowledge, to set it, to bring the parts into as good contact as you possibly can ; then look to the Great Healer for a good recovery. Should you sit down with one bone in one direction and another at a different angle, and ask God to cure? As well go about without shoes and stockings, and ask God to protect you that your feet may not be injured. But you meet with cases where medical skill is unavailing—then pray."

The condition of the medical school, while a source of encouragement to the Doctor, called forth occasionally the exercise of rare tact and wisdom.

"The Viceroy left the young men entirely under my charge," he writes, "and at first I had a good deal of trouble ; on one occasion the fellows mutinied. The difficulty was this, they mistook kindness for weakness, and thought that as I spoke to them about their spiritual state they could act as they pleased ! I have had to learn how difficult it is to seek the salvation of those for whose discipline you are responsible. Finally, however, in God's mercy and in answer to prayer, the matter is now definitely settled. The students have a prayer-meeting every morning amongst themselves, and although it is quite optional, about twelve out of eighteen attend it now. It is conducted in turn by four of the men themselves. On Sunday afternoon we have a Bible class, which all are required to attend.

"A little while ago one of the Christians brought in the captain of a torpedo launch to see me, who had received his education in America. The student had been speaking and praying with him, and begged me to speak to the young officer about his soul. I found him trusting in Christ as his Saviour. He had recently passed through a lot of trouble, having met with a collision at sea, and was in Tien-tsin during the trial of the case. He had come under the influence of some of his friends in the medical school, and appeared to be soundly converted.

"Only last Friday we had a special meeting amongst the students, because there seemed to be a good deal of the spirit of prayer present, and although it was perfectly optional, every student was present, besides two friends. We had a delightful time reading and talking about the eighth chapter of Romans, together with prayer and the singing of Sankey's hymns. The men know now that if they do wrong the necessary punishment will follow; but, thank God, I have very, very seldom to interfere.

" Might I ask your earnest prayers for the hospital
and medical school? What rich blessings would
come down if our friends at home made particular
matters in the Mission field subjects of prayer, and
so fulfilled the Word of our blessed Lord, Matt. xviii.
19. I am sure our Father would fulfil His portion.
I have been thinking a good deal lately whether
something might not be done in this matter. I have
seen such blessed results follow in answer to direct
and pointed believing prayer, that I should like to
send home to friends the names of individual Chinese,
if they would insert them in their praying lists.
Suppose two friends took one or two names, making
use of the promise above quoted. I would agree to
keep track of the individual prayed for. If some
dear brethren and sisters in England were thus
engaged, they would be working distinctly for the
Chinese,—the names given being those who have
had, or are getting, Christian instruction. What do
you think of this? Anyhow, I will send you six
names, and especially I ask prayer for myself. If
this plan could only be arranged (and any number
of names could be given if friends were only forthcoming), we might have Christians who could not
leave England, yet in active work for the conversion
of the Chinese. For we want more direct, intelligent
prayer, not vague requests."

During the summer of this year, 1885, Dr.
Mackenzie was laid low with what it was at first
feared would prove a most serious illness. He had

for many years suffered from attacks of malarial
fever, and at this time he was attacked by heat apo-
plexy, and lost, for some hours, the use of his right
hand and the power of speech. Upon his recovery
it was seen to be absolutely necessary that he should
seek change of air, and his friends Mr. and Mrs.
Hobson, of the Customs Service, who were at that
time contemplating a visit to Taku, at the mouth
of the Peiho, thoughtfully arranged to have an additional native house-boat lashed to the side of their
own for the Doctor's use, and in their genial companionship he spent several weeks, benefiting greatly
by the rest and change.

"A community of pilots reside here," writes the
Doctor to his father, "who take steamers in and out
over the bar. The place is very flat and muddy, and
its only attraction is its neighbourhood to the sea
and the fact of the air being consequently pure. I
am much stronger for my stay of a week. I have
been twice over the bar in a tug, and as this is a
distance of seven miles, one gets a really good blow.
Dear little Maggie will be a great comfort to you.
Child-life is so helpful to us ; we little know how much
joy we derive from companionship with children, not
perhaps until we lose it. During my residence in
Taku I have been living among children, and their
sweet voices around one are full of the best music."

At about this time one of the Doctor's students
became seriously ill, and it was considered necessary
that he should have a change of air. Accompanied

by a companion, he went down to Taku with the
Doctor in another house-boat. A letter written at
this time by the young medical student who acted as
nurse to his sick friend is an interesting proof of Dr.
Mackenzie's influence over these educated young
Chinamen.

"One of my fellow-students had been suffering
from malarial fever," he writes, "before Dr. Mackenzie's
illness, and his temperature increased to 105° Fahr.
He was then advised to take a trip down to Taku,
and I went with and took care of him.

"The Doctor had one house-boat, Mr. Hobson one,
and we one. It took us a day and a half to go down
to our destination. The Doctor and Mr. Hobson
landed at Taku and lived at one of the captains', but
we stayed on the boat, for my patient wished to get
the sea-breezes. I might have had a jolly time then
if I had not been so lonesome and yoked with care.
It needs a great deal of patience to attend to a patient.
But more than this, one evening after the sun had
set, all of a sudden dark clouds spread over the sky,
the north-easterly wind blew violently, and it rained
copiously. We were all terribly frightened. Then I
prayed to the Lord our Saviour, who alone hath
power over the wind, and we sang the holy hymn,
'Peace, be still.' Afterwards I had peace within
from above, though there was trouble without. How
God wrought in me I could not exactly tell, but it
was so. We got through the tempest safe and sound,
under the shelter of the protecting wings of our

loving Father in heaven. About a fortnight ago we returned to the hospital, and my friend is now convalescent; but I have been attacked by the same type of fever. While I was lying ill the books you were so kind as to send down were read to me by some of my friends here, and I delighted very much to hear them.

"I know that our faith is indeed small, but God increaseth it by our earnest and fervent prayers, and I have experienced that no matter where we may be, or whatever troubles or dangers may come to us, our kind Heavenly Father is willing and able to take care of us, if we only trust in Him."

Another of the medical students, writing to the same friend a short time after, speaks of the illness of his fellow-students and the Doctor, and tells how when the invalids left Tien-tsin, they formed an evening prayer-meeting to pray for them and for their friends in China and other lands.

"We know that our prayers are answered, and will be by no means in vain," writes the young student. "We hope that our faith in Christ will grow stronger day by day. We know that when our term of three years is expired we shall be put either into camp or men-of-war, where we are liable to be surrounded by temptation and evil ones. How can we expect ourselves to be able to stand this? we are so young It is a rather hard thing. However, we will cast ourselves in the hand of the Almighty, and pray to Him for help and strength. We must imitate St.

Paul, who says, 'I can do all things through Christ, which strengtheneth me.'"

After speaking of a journey Dr. Mackenzie undertook at this time, he continues :—

"The Doctor is hoping that he may go into the interior oftener; but, in fact, it is very hard for him to leave us. He does not feel comfortable without teaching us something every day. I can see the way in which he treats us. He is exceedingly kind to us, and I hope God will spare our lives to finish our course of study, and do something for the Chinese Government, and, finally, we may find some way or other to repay the Doctor's great kindness. I am very grateful for his teaching. I cannot express all my thoughts and thanks to him, for my knowledge is so limited."

Dr. Mackenzie's Bible classes were always found to be most helpful by those who had the privilege of attending them, the secret of his success doubtless lying in the fact that it was always his aim to make these meetings as conversational as possible, and to induce as many of the members to take part as he possibly could.

"People enjoy a meeting much more when they have some part in it, however small," he once wrote. "Above all things, the leader should avoid preaching, if the meeting is to be interesting and profitable."

Extracts from Dr. Mackenzie's note-book with regard to these classes show how fully his practice agreed with this theory, and how thorough an interest the Chinese members of his classes showed in the subjects of their lessons.

"We were talking to-day upon the text, ' Blessed are ye that hunger now,' " he writes, " and I asked, ' How is it that there are so few that hunger after spiritual things?' 'Why,' replied one of the Chinese Christians, ' it is for this reason, I think : when a man is sick he won't feel hungry at sight of the best dinner you can put before him : his disease must be cured before he can feel hungry. And so it is with spiritual things : this disease of sin must be grappled with before we can begin to feel hungry for heavenly things.' On another occasion we were reading of how Jesus, while preaching by the Lake of Gennesaret, being troubled by the crowds which pressed upon Him, sought refuge in a fishing-boat belonging to Simon Peter, and it is stated that at the time the fishermen were engaged in washing their nets. ' Ah !' remarked young Mao, one of our Christian dispensers, ' we want to imitate Peter in this. He and his fellow-disciples had toiled all night and caught nothing, and here they were found in the morning washing their nets. We, who are fishers of men, need to attend to this ; we should be washing our nets oftener. Are we not succeeding in our work as we should like? Perhaps our communion with the Saviour is broken. Perhaps we are not constantly feeding upon God's Word. Then are our nets foul, and we had better give up fishing until we have washed our nets.' "

The Doctor also gives many interesting incidents in connection with his medical students' Bible class, showing that many of the young men took a deep interest in spiritual things. It was not wonderful that an earnest desire after higher attainments in the Divine life should be tested, and an attempt made to hinder spiritual growth by the great enemy of souls. An account of some of the trials through which they had to pass is given by Dr. Mackenzie in a letter of this period.

" One student, who had given a good deal of trouble, had to be punished for flagrant disobedience ; so he worked up some of the younger men, and got them to go to the yamen of the Taotai, the next official in rank here to the Viceroy, complaining of one of the assistant-teachers ; and, to back up their case, one of them took a Bible with him, and pulled it out before the official, declaring that I taught them more Christianity than medicine.

" Of course this was a falsehood, as no Christian teaching is allowed to interfere with their medical classes, excepting on Sundays, when medical class work is suspended, and I hold a Bible class instead. Well, the effect of this appeal was that the Taotai gave them a good rating, and though he was not a Christian, publicly told them that he knew what Christian work I was doing amongst them was for their good, and sent them back under an escort. The end of it has been that the ringleader was dismissed from the school, and the others would have been punished, but I begged them off, as they were all repentant.

"Our Bible class and Sabbath keeping, which was before carried out upon my sole responsibility, has now had official sanction, with the request only that those who did not wish to attend should not be compelled, but should instead carry on their medical studies as usual on the Sundays. One after another, however, begged to be allowed to attend again, and now all but one are coming voluntarily. One young fellow pleaded the case of the prodigal. 'When the younger son came back the father forgave him, even though he had been bad, did he not?' he enquired. Another told me he 'was not very religious, but he did believe in Christianity.' Of course one was only too glad to receive the poor fellows back again."

CHAPTER XIII.

STRANGE PHASES OF CHINESE LIFE.

CHAPTER XIII.

STRANGE PHASES OF CHINESE LIFE.

FROM his earliest days in China Dr. Mackenzie had always felt a deep interest in work among the people of the villages and country towns. He had a strong belief that the gospel would take a firmer hold on these simple folks, and that its greatest triumphs would be won there rather than in the thickly-populated centres of trade and commerce. It has already been noticed that he had frequently desired to pay visits to the country stations, but had found himself tied to his all-absorbing work in the hospital and medical school. He had hoped that the Viceroy would be willing to appoint another foreign medical man to assist him in his laborious work of training students for the Chinese Government ; but His Excellency did not care to entertain the idea, although he allowed two of the Doctor's former pupils to be retained as assistants by him. But now that the Hospital Reserve Fund was steadily growing and bringing in an increasing yearly income, Dr. Mackenzie began to cherish a hope that from that source it would be practicable to support an additional medical

277

missionary to the Tien-tsin station, who should not only be able to share with him the duties connected with the hospital and medical school, but whose presence would also enable them alternately to pay frequent visits to the country stations, and so increase and strengthen the work there.

In the autumn of 1885 he wrote to the Directors, urging them to seek for and send out an additional medical missionary.

"Is there no way of making our needs known to the Christian medical men of London, Edinburgh, and Cambridge?" he enquires. "There was a revival among the students of Edinburgh and Cambridge resulting from the 'Stanley Smith movement.' Many medical professors and senior students engaged in evangelistic tours as the result, and the missionary spirit spread extensively. Is there no way of reaching them? Would not a paragraph in such a paper as *The Christian* be likely to catch the attention of such men? I think so.

"Last month I had to take a health change, so I went with Mr. Lees and Mr. Bryson on a visit to our stations at Yen-Shan and Ching-yün.

"I have always been a firm believer in country work, from what I have seen of the country people who come into the hospital. I was delighted with our visit. We have no paid agent at present in this district, yet there are quite a large number of converts, who are holding on in their profession with such simple trust, that it is a pleasure to meet with them and to hear them pray. Yet the ignorance is vast ; take one village, for instance, in which there are perhaps twenty converts, and yet not one of them can read or write. They meet together to sing, knowing a few of Sankey's hymns by heart, and they pray and exhort each other. How great is their need of a teacher ! The possibilities of extension in this region I believe to be vast. The people outside the converts are kindly disposed, and appear willing to learn. I took a few medicines with me, but the demand was far beyond what I could supply, as crowds came flocking in from all regions. Now this hopeful district is visited twice a year by the foreign missionary, who spends two or three days there each time. Had we but another medical missionary in Tien-tsin I could get away twice a year, and thus four visits instead of two could be paid. It would be quite possible, too, to establish in time one or two branch dispensaries in this region, in charge of trained natives, who could be evangelist and doctor in one ; but it would be useless to attempt it unless properly supervised by the foreign missionary."

In connection with this visit Dr. Mackenzie relates a story illustrating the perseverance, under persecution, of a woman who became interested in the gospel, and who lived in this district. " Her mother-in-law strongly objected to her learning the doctrine, and tried to prevent her attendance at Mrs. Fan's instruction class. Finally, the old woman told her if she went to the Bible-woman's house again she would lock her out. She was accustomed to go in the evening, after the day's work was done. Mrs. Fan, the Bible-woman, lived near by in another court, which communicated by a lane with the court in which the young woman lived. One evening, as usual, she attended the meeting, but on returning found the gate leading from the lane into her court locked. She could not get past, so she went back and borrowed a ladder, and by its aid climbed on to the roof of the neighbouring house, which was of course single-storied. She pulled up the ladder, dragged it over the roof of the house, and let it down on the other side, and so descended. She continued this manner of returning home night after night for a considerable time, and finally her mother-in-law also became a believer in Jesus."

In January 1886, in consequence of the large number of deaths constantly occurring in the Tien-tsin foundling hospital, the Taotai requested Dr. Mackenzie kindly to inspect the institution, and try and discover the cause of the great mortality among the infants.

" The institution is supported by the salt guilds of the city," writes Dr. Mackenzie, " and they allow tls. 600 per month for its support. I found three hundred and ten children, all girls, in the building. One wet nurse is allowed to two children. They live in rooms opening on to a court, and sleep on the brick beds, where the women's food is cooked. In all the rooms there were only windows on one side, and

these were closely papered. In one apartment, about
twenty-two feet by ten, with kangs on three sides, were
eight women and sixteen children. The rooms were
very dirty and very close, and cooking utensils and dirty
rags were lying about freely. There was an enormous
amount of eye disease ; probably every third child
had bad eyes. Not a child cried, but all sat stupid,
and dosed in the arms of the women, one on each
arm. They were no doubt all drugged. The place
was managed by head amahs, old women, who talked
tremendously. ' Do they never cry ? ' I enquired of a
head amah, who has two children to look after. ' Oh
no, they are so well cared for ! ' she replied.

" Officials robed in silks, satins, and furs, with embroidered garments and precious stones,—nine persons
in all, two of them Taotais,—inspect these dirty buildings, and a mandarin's lady comes once a month for
the same purpose. The Customs Taotai thinks instead of good harm is being done."

In his hospital work the Doctor not unfrequently
encountered curious phases of Chinese life. He mentions the case of one patient who was a great athlete,
said to be able to lift a man into the air with one
hand. In order to conserve and increase his strength,
according to Chinese theory, he had not slept lying
down for twenty years. At first he could only sit up
half the night, but at the present time finds it easier
to sleep sitting up than lying down. He leans his
head forward against his arms on the wall or window,
and so sleeps."

On another occasion the Doctor was called to see a man lying in his coffin, on a piece of waste land behind the hospital. It was supposed that he had died, and a coffin having been procured, according to common Chinese custom, the body was placed in it and put out upon the plain, instead of being interred,—the usual practice being to bury after a longer or shorter period, often many months elapsing between the day of death and the day of entombment.

A man walking on the plain next morning fancied he heard a rustle inside the coffin ; standing still, he heard the noise repeated. In a short time a curious crowd had collected ; the lid was removed, and the man was found to be still alive.

Water was given to him, and he drank it. Dr. Mackenzie was sent for, and when he saw the man he was breathing quietly, but still unconscious, and he ordered him brandy and milk.

At this time he writes to his father :—

" I am very fully occupied, for which indeed I am exceedingly thankful. I will tell you how I am spending my time.

" My hour to rise in the morning is half-past six for winter, breakfast at a quarter to eight. At a quarter past eight I conduct a sort of Bible class in the hospital among the patients (those who are able to come), and the dispensers and servants. This lasts for three-quarters of an hour, and is, of course, in Chinese. From half-past nine till eleven o'clock I study Chinese ; at eleven o'clock dispensary work begins, and here and in the hospital I spend two hours, until one o'clock. At one o'clock I take dinner ; at two prepare my medical class work ; at three I take the senior class in the medical school in medicine or surgery ; at four or half-past four I am free, and I try to get away for a walk, but there is constantly something coming up to be attended to— perhaps an operation, or a Chinese letter to answer, or some case of discipline in the medical school to be dealt with.

"On Tuesday evenings at seven p.m. we have a Chinese prayer-meeting, with a review of the week's work in the Bible ; this I conduct. On Monday even- ing we have a Mission prayer-meeting, when we all meet for consultation and prayer. On Wednesday evening there is the Union Church prayer-meeting, which is practically a united missionary prayer- meeting, and which I always attend.

"Sunday is also a very busy day. Sunday-school class at half-past nine ; Chinese service at half-past ten ; medical school Bible class at three p.m. ; evening service at six p.m. ; meeting for 'Blue-jackets,' from English and American navy, after the evening service in the church.

"There, I did not know what to write about, so I thought it might interest you to hear how I get along from day to day. I feel what a privilege it is to be doing God's work among the Chinese. There is a good deal of seed sowing, of course, but it is work that has to be done by some one, and we are continually cheered by seeing the good seed springing up and bringing forth fruit. Our loving Saviour is indeed a good Master to serve."

The Sunday afternoon Bible class for medical students, to which reference has been made, was not confined to these young men alone, but other foreign friends outside the Mission circle were in the habit of attending it, and felt it a great stimulus to their spiritual life. He had also a class in the Chinese Sunday-school, which met, at that time, at half-past nine, before the morning service. He took great interest in his Chinese scholars, all of whom were grown-up men, and not children, as is usually the case at home.

In his diary he mentions one man who became a Sunday scholar, and afterwards a patient. He seems to have been brought to the class by one who had long been a member of it, and was a true believer, though his knowledge was very small. We would fain hope his case is a typical one, and that there may be many other Chinese disciples, poor, unknown, and with little courage, and yet known of God, as the day shall reveal.

Chang-yü-ch'wen, the keeper of one of the public buildings of Tien-tsin, had been for many years a Christian, and was a member of the Doctor's Sunday-school class. He observed for some days in succession a man engaged in picking up stray bits of rag and paper in the neighbourhood of the hall, and entered into conversation with him. He found the rag-picker at first somewhat reserved in his manners, and in answer to the common Chinese question, " How much money do you make daily by this work ? " he replied indefinitely, " Oh, enough to live upon." But Chang felt his interest in the man aroused, and continuing the conversation, by-and-bye discovered that the stranger, who also bore the common Chinese name of Chang, was about forty years of age, and had land in the country belonging to him. " Why are you away from home then ? " was the natural enquiry. Oh, he had left home because his family persecuted him so, and would give him no rest. " Why, how is that ? " " I was going to the meetings of a religious sect, and they tried to stop me ; then, because I would not stop going, they were constantly swearing at and tormenting me in every way. At last they would give me no food to eat. I am not a member of the Church of which I speak ; I am only a believer in its doctrines. Finally, I felt I could bear it no longer, so I decided to leave home just as I was, without any money, so that I could escape from their persecution." " Can you read ? " asked Chang. " No, not a character." " Have you learnt the catechism ? " " No, but I know that I am a sinner, and I have heard that the Lord can save me, and I believe." " Why ! " exclaimed Yü-Ch'wen, " I am a believer too ; I am a Christian. You should come with me to our church on Sundays." And so the stranger was brought to the Sunday-school class, and became an attentive listener to the Doctor's earnest words.

In future conversations it was discovered that the man had a friend in Tien-tsin, a neighbour from his own country-side, and this friend had offered him a situation, with his food and a yearly wage. But the wanderer would not take it ; he said he "had some occupation," but his real reason for refusing the offer was that he feared he would not be able to attend church if he accepted it, and he was afraid to confess that he was a Christian. Some time after this friend found the man out again, and repeated his offer of the post. This time he ventured to say that he would take the situation if he might have four days a month to attend to a private matter ; but this was immediately refused, and the friend departed.

He makes, by picking up paper, sufficient to keep himself in food and lodging, and seems quite satisfied. Pointing to the rich and well-dressed people passing in large numbers along the Taku Road, Yû Ch'wen asked him one day if he was not surprised that he should be left so poor, while others had all they needed. "Ah," replied the man, "this life is not for ever." ,

Later on he fell sick, and was brought to the hospital, suffering from dysentery. He stayed for a few days, but as there was no marked improvement in his symptoms, he asked permission to leave, wishing to be treated after Chinese methods. Some days later his death was reported in a poor Chinese inn. He was not a man of strong courage, but he had readily given up his all for freedom to worship the Lord in whom he believed.

In May 1886 the Doctor mentions, in his diary, the case of a man who had been that morning baptized. He came into the hospital nearly blind, and great improvement followed upon operation. He returned home trusting in the Lord Jesus, but not baptized. His first act upon arriving at his village was to take down the idols in his home, and throw them into a neighbouring pond. His conduct was so strange that the people thought he was mad, and called him so. After many months he came back to Tien-tsin to receive baptism. Two months after being received into the Church, he returned again from his village, apparently as earnest as ever. It seems that he is often overcome in arguments with his neighbours, because his knowledge is so slight.

As an illustration of the curious modes of treatment in vogue among Chinese doctors, I select a few cases mentioned in Dr. Mackenzie's note-book, the results of his own experience.

" I was called in to see a child, six months of age, at one of the yamens. It was suffering from bronchitis. A large toad, with its belly in contact with the child's body, had been employed, the claws being covered with cotton wool, the object being to draw away the heat. Scorpions had also been cooked and made into a poultice, which was applied to the fontanel of the infant. The stings were made into a broth, and the child fed with it."

Another patient he mentions as having been treated for typhoid fever at home. The doctor applied burn-

ing incense to a piece of leaf laid on the skin. The
leaf was set on fire, and burnt the skin. Many years
after, over a hundred scars were visible on his body
as the result of this treatment.

Still another case was that of a man suffering from
severe dyspepsia, and very much reduced. He said
he had experienced slight discomfort, but was quite
strong a month ago, when he consulted a priest-
doctor, who stuck six needles into his gastric region,
after which treatment he had to keep his bed for a
month, and could eat nothing but slops.

" I was called to attend a woman in one of the
yamens, who was suffering from spasmodic asthma,
and found a slave-girl beating the back of the chest
with a large stick like a rolling-pin, with the idea of
giving relief."

The Doctor's diary contains many instances of
Chinese customs which seem strange and often cruel
to us. Among others, he notes the practice of laying
out a person who is dying before the decease takes
place.

" A Chinese friend of mine had an uncle, aged
sixty-four, who has been ill for some time past, and
the other day they sent him word the old man was
dying and had been laid out. In China, when all
hope is given up of a patient's recovery, the custom
is to dress them at once in grave clothes, and remove
them to a board and tressels away from the ordinary
bed, so that it shall not be defiled. As it is often
uncertain when a man is going to breathe his last,

it not unfrequently happens that his last hours are spent in torture, and his end hastened by this treatment. In the cold winter of Tien-tsin, to be stripped of warm garments and bedding and laid out in cold, stiff clothing must indeed be trying.

"My friend arrived at his uncle's house, expecting to find him dead, but instead of this he was only laid out in burial clothes; he was surrounded by a crowd of relatives, dressed in white mourning garments, waiting for him to breathe his last, while strips of white paper, the sign of death in a house, had already been pasted on the outer doors. 'Do you know me?' my friend asked of his dying uncle. 'Oh yes; why did you not come before?' replied the patient; 'I am so thirsty, and they will give me nothing to drink, and I am so cold, since all my warm clothing has been taken away, and my bones are sore with lying on this hard board. Move me back to the kang, and take these clothes away; I am not dead yet!' The nephew gave him a bowl of hot water, which he drank, and afterwards some tea. He felt his pulse, and discovered that it was stronger than when he had visited him before.

"'Don't wait for me, father!' said a married daughter who had just arrived; 'I am here, so you can go!' This remark was made in allusion to the idea that the souls of the dying cannot pass away if they are desiring to see some absent member of the family.

"The Christian nephew insisted upon his uncle being moved back to his bed and dressed again in

19

warm clothing, and gave him some arrowroot; after which the old man seemed better, and lived for about a fortnight."

At about the same time the Doctor writes :—

" Here is an instance of the domestic misery so often found in this heathen land. A man had been attending our dispensary for several weeks, suffering from a very painful and incurable malady, for which, however, we could give him much relief. One day his wife appeared with him, and wished to know whether he could be permanently cured. Finding that this was impossible, she began to upbraid her poor husband for his inability to work, and, finally, turning to me in the presence of the sick man, asked if I would not give him a dose of poison to kill him quickly, as they had to depend for their support upon the labour of one son."

In July of this year Dr. Mackenzie writes to his brother :—

" I have been away for a boat trip of ten days' duration, to try and shake off my malaria this summer, and so prevent breaking down as I did last year. We are very badly situated in Tien-tsin for getting a change, having no hills near and no seaside resort nearer than Chefoo.

" Determined to get some sort of a change, I went with Mr. King on this boat trip to one of our country stations. The journey, however, was rather a mistake, as in a small boat, with a little cabin, it was unbearably hot.

" After the sun had been on the boat for some hours, we were in a state of agony, endeavouring in every way to cool ourselves, sitting with wet towels round our heads and chests.   It was a dreadful time ; yet upon our return I feel the better for even such a trying change ; the air, free from the neighbourhood of a great city, was at least pure, and I feel freer from the depressing languor of the malarial atmosphere of this place."

" A Tauist priest came to the hospital to-day," he writes, " with his right ear badly deformed.   Two and a half years ago, when his temple needed repairing, he himself nailed both his ears to a door, and remained thus for two days and two nights. His object was to excite compassion and stimulate liberality.   In freeing himself one ear, the right, got badly torn, and has since remained hanging as an awkward fragment.   The left ear, though torn through, had healed in good position."

In the autumn of 1886 it was decided to try and form all the medical missionaries in China, both men and women, into a society, to be known as the " Medical Missionary Association of China."   It was also arranged that a journal should be started by this society, to be called the *Medical Missionary Journal.* It is an interesting proof of the estimation in which Dr. Mackenzie was held by his colleagues in medical work, that he was chosen by them to edit the part of this magazine which was to be devoted to the consideration of the best methods of using medical

missionary work as a means of doing the Master's
work and saving souls.

Dr. Mackenzie's time had always been so fully
occupied that it had seemed almost impossible for
him to use his pen in describing the wonderful work
he was privileged to carry on, or to express in writing
his ideas of a medical missionary's calling.   This
work being almost entirely supported by the liberality
of the Viceroy, there was not the same need of
writing a report for the encouragement and interest
of foreign contributions as exists in many other cases.
But when this journal was started, he seemed to look
upon this appointment as a call coming, first of all,
from the Master ; and during the last fifteen months
of his life, the period of the magazine's existence, he
contributed to it repeatedly.

" The Evangelistic Side of a Medical Mission," and
" Some Spiritual Results of Medical Mission Work,"
were the titles of two of these papers, and an editorial
called " The Double Cure," which appeared within
a few weeks of his death, and was his last contribution
to the pages of the periodical, speaks with no uncertain
sound of the aim which Kenneth Mackenzie kept
ever in view in the prosecution of his medical work.

CHAPTER XIV.

GLIMPSES OF INNER LIFE.

CHAPTER XIV.

GLIMPSES OF INNER LIFE.

IT has been before mentioned that Dr. Mackenzie constantly acknowledged his indebtedness for assistance in hospital work to the medical men of the Tien-tsin community, Drs. Frazer and Irwin, and also to the surgeons of the various gunboats which, during the winter, are usually stationed in Tien-tsin, besides those medical missionaries coming down from the interior, and residing in the port for a time.

" I have had a very pleasant associate this summer," writes the Doctor, " in Dr. Merritt from Pao-ting-fu, who has been spending the summer here, with his family ; he has given me great help every day in my work. It is very enjoyable to have companions who are interested in just the same line of things as one-self. I have been very busy this summer, but greatly enjoy the work. I get now an increasingly large amount of surgical work, and generally have two or three important operations every week-day. Eye operations are of almost daily occurrence, and it is a real pleasure to restore sight to those who come to us, to all intents and purposes, blind. I feel I should like to be relieved of the teaching work in my hands.

I am afraid I did not count the cost when I started with it.. It is a tremendous tax upon one, the constant preparation for class work in the midst of so many practical hospital duties, and is especially felt during the hot months of summer. Not that I do not enjoy it too, and shall ever feel grateful for the privilege of, in some measure, influencing the lives of a few of the first representatives of Western medicine, as practised by the Chinese themselves. Still it is a strain I would not like to bear alone much longer. I have very efficient Chinese helpers from my old classes, but they can never quite take the place of foreign associates. But this is too much about self and his doings."

Towards the end of December Dr. Mackenzie writes to his brother from Peking :—

"You will see that I have left home. I came away two days before Christmas, with Mr. Gilmour, who had visited Tien-tsin from Mongolia to get some drugs from me. I thought a little change into another region would do me good, and I was able to get Dr. Leach, of the American gunboat *Palos*, to take on my work during my absence ; so I came away with Gilmour. He is a delightful companion, and though the journey to Peking, at this time of the year, is rather trying, I greatly enjoyed it. We travelled by cart, as the river is frozen, starting about 9 a.m., and reaching our inn about 7 p.m. Then we had a meal, and slept on the brick bed until 3 a.m., when we had to get up and continue our journey during the night. This part of it was very cold at this season. We again travelled most of the Friday night, and were thus able to get in at 8 a.m. on Christmas morning. Every one was very kind, and welcomed us heartily.

"I have been spending these days in social visits amongst my friends in Peking, who are so very kind. Yesterday I was lunching with Dr. Atterbury, and was glad to see something of him and his work. You will perhaps remember that it was he who came down to Tien-tsin to take up my work during my absence in England. I shall ever remember this act of kindness. He has just completed a fine new hospital for Medical Mission work, built at his own cost.

"Depend upon it, there are not a few unselfish people in the world, who live, not for themselves, but for others. In these cases wealth is a rich blessing.

"I am very glad to know more of Gilmour. Living away in Mongolia, he sees no foreign face, and no fellow-countryman is there to sympathize with him. He has no house of his own, and, living in the miserable inns of the place, knows nothing of privacy, for the Chinese and Mongols, according to custom, crowd around him at all hours. He takes simple medicines that I make up for him, and opens a booth on the street, where he gives away his medicines and preaches the gospel to those who come around him. It is a hard life, but God has given him much grace and strength to bear it."

A fortnight after he writes :—

" I stayed in Peking over the week of prayer, and the meetings every day were delightful. I got to know all the missionaries in Peking. Previously I have been kept so closely to my work in Tien-tsin that I only knew many of them by name, or in a casual way ; now I can say I know most of them as a friend knows his friend.

" I was received in Peking by all the friends with such unbounded kindness, that I cannot but praise the Lord for all His goodness to me. We had most blessed meetings, and the spirit of prayer was poured forth in such rich abundance, that it is evident God is about to do a great work in North China this year. I hope Maggie is keeping well. I wish I could see the dear child now and again, and visit you all ; yet I am far from being unhappy, God has given me rich joy in my life-work. I know that I am doing work for God here in Tien-tsin. The hospital is one of the most important centres of usefulness in the whole of China. It amazes me sometimes as I look back, to see how wonderfully out of a small beginning God has developed a large and efficient institution. We seek ever to bring home the precious gospel of the love of God to our patients in hospital, so that from this centre the Truth is carried away for hundreds of miles."

Writing to a medical friend in China, soon after his return from Peking, Dr. Mackenzie says :—

" I am more and more impressed with the fact that it is useless for us to pray for an outpouring of the

Holy Spirit upon the people amongst whom we live and labour, unless we are earnestly seeking His presence ourselves. I am sure of this, that God works through His people. Glory be to His holy Name that it is so! If the people are to get the Holy Spirit, we must first seek it for ourselves, and then, when we are filled, the Spirit will, like a great stream that has overflown its banks, pour forth to others; or else (God grant that it may not be so in our experience) He will pass us by, and use some other of His servants. But the appointed channel of His blessing is through His spiritual Church in its various members. We are to be co-workers with God, and yet after all the whole work is His; we need but to be willing and empty. But oh, how much is implied in this. 'Hungering and thirsting after righteousness,' 'Travailing in soul'—these are some of the expressions in the Word to denote the state of heart of him whom God can richly bless and use. This is no Sunday religion, dear brother, but a life full of the healthiest activities and most ennobling joys."

Dr. Mackenzie's time was so fully occupied that he had little leisure for reading, and, with the exception of professional literature, during the latter years of his life read only books and papers which he considered helpful to personal piety, such as Andrew Murray's "Abide in Christ," "Like Christ," and others of the same series; "The Life of Finney," 'The Christian and the Reaper."

Some time before this date he had written to his father :—

" I am glad you have enjoyed ' Abide in Christ ; ' it is a book full of rich teaching.   I think I have hardly ever received more benefit from any book.   It requires much careful thought.   I get very little time for general reading, but such a book as this can be taken up at odd intervals, and fill the mind with food for meditation."

To a Christian friend, connected with the Chinese customs service, who was at home on furlough, he wrote, under date of March 1887, thanking him for a book he had received, and continued :—

" I am looking forward to having a great treat in reading it.   At present I am still feasting on ' Like Christ,' and also another little book entitled ' Thoughts on Christian Sanctity,' by Rev. H. C. G. Moule.   This latter book I am sure you would like, if you have not already read it.   You see, I haven't much time for general reading, and these books, to be of any benefit, must be assimilated, and this is a slow process. Gilmour came in from Mongolia at the New Year, and I let him take with him ' Abide in Christ.' . . . . I have already got rid of half-a-dozen copies.

" Oh, dear brother, it is a precious thing to serve the Lord.   I have never known such joy in life as God has mercifully granted me these last few months. Jesus literally fills and satisfies one's life.   It is such a pleasure to see the students growing in knowledge of God.   The dear Saviour will indeed reveal Himself in His glory to us (Chinaman or foreigner) if we will but get near enough to see Him.

"You will remember —— and ——; they are at home on furlough after their three years' course. The former has met with a lot of persecution from his relatives because he has become a Christian, but the Lord is sustaining him, and causing him to bear witness for Jesus. He writes from his home that he would 'rather die than deny Christ.' Then —— is preaching and holding Bible classes in his holidays, and has already led some to the Cross.

"In the hospital there is a good work going on ; the Lord Jesus seems to be working all the time amongst our in-patients. We are having enquirers always ; that is, no sooner is one batch gone than another has taken its place. Last year there was an average of forty in-patients all the time in the wards ; out of this number we always have some who are seeking the Lord, and give evidence of having the Holy Spirit in their hearts. This is a great joy to us."

After relating the case of a man who had come into he hospital a heathen, in total ignorance of the gospel, and had died full of joy in hope of salvation through our Lord and Saviour, he continues :—

"Yes, indeed, St. Paul knew what he was about when he wrote, 'The gospel of Christ is the power of God unto salvation to every one that believeth.'

"This winter has been an unusually worldly one

in Tien-tsin. They have had the municipal band playing at the skating rink on Sundays regularly, besides Sunday hunting.

" This is largely due to the influence of a growing French and German element. What a sad spectacle it is, while the Chinese are entering the Kingdom, to see men and women from Christian lands trampling under foot the precious gospel, and ashamed of it. Yet so it was with the Jews, God's chosen people. Oh to walk before Him with fear and trembling, that we slip not ! "

To another friend, a young missionary in China, with whom he frequently corresponded, he writes :—

" The first year in China is always a trying time, because it is a time of preparation, and we yearn to be doing. When you have got some hold of the language, and can engage in work for the Master, you will have your hands and your heart full. And yet, even now, you are actively working for the Lord. To do the work that lies at our hands, this is fulfilling God's will. If I were you I would not touch medicine for at least a year, but give your whole strength to the language and to looking after your own health. Medical missionaries are usually forced into medical work from the beginning, and then have to lament it ever after. Get a good foundation laid in the language, and take plenty of exercise in the open air.

" You mention that in leaving England you fear you will lose much religious teaching. I do trust it will not be so. I am learning that public religious services are after all but imperfect methods of giving religious instruction—I mean heart instruction. The greatest help I find in the Christian life is in the prayerful study of the Bible. John vi. 57 is a striking verse, 'As I live by the Father, so he that eateth Me, even he shall live by Me.' Our Lord, it seems to me, would have us learn that exactly the same sort of relationship which existed between the Man Christ Jesus, and the Father in heaven, is open to us. He was ever depending upon the help of the Father, was ever seeking to obey the Father, and was in the closest communion with the Father. We can only live as fruitful branches when we are in vital contact with the Vine. We can only become and remain in vital contact by eating of Him, partaking of His life ; and this spiritual food can only be obtained direct from Jesus. I fall into temptation when I get up late in the morning, and lose my communion with God over His Word. Nothing, no united service, or even family prayers, can take the place of this. Studying God's Word upon one's knees I have found the most helpful of all methods. How willing the Lord is to come and dwell in us if we only want Him ! And then if He is dwelling in us, the world wears a different aspect, and we are very rarely long in doubt as to our course of action in any matter."

To the same friend, at a later date, after a family bereavement, he writes :—

"It is a terrible calamity to lose a loved parent ;

yet the loss is ours only, and we should not sorrow
as those who have no hope.   Dying is but 'going
home' to the believer ; for has not our blessed
Lord abolished death, and brought life and immor-
tality to light through the gospel?   Let us just dwell
upon the verse, for there is no more death to those
who are in Christ Jesus.   It is but the coming to the
end of our earthly journey, and entering into the
Promised Land.   The verse rings of victory.   What
a joy that you have found Christ so precious to you
of late !   He will bear the pain for you, and in
bringing it to Him you will learn to know Him better,
for is it not in sorrow and trouble that our dearest
friendships are made, that we come nearer to our
friends?   He is our Friend.

"Let me give you a verse that has been full of comfort to me (Phil. iv. 6) ' In nothing be anxious ; but in
everything by prayer and supplication with thanksgiving, let your requests be made known unto God.'
Verse 7, ' And the peace of God, which passeth all
understanding, shall guard your hearts and your
thoughts in Christ Jesus.'   Verse 7 contains one of the
most precious promises in the Bible.   Just think of
having His wonderful peace guarding one's heart and
one's thoughts all day long.   But it is only on condition
that we fulfil the sixth verse.   ' In nothing be anxious,'
—this is a distinct command, and if we fail to fulfil it
we shall not get the blessing.   Sorrow even is anxiety,
and should be laid upon our blessed Lord.   Then in
prayer and supplication we must not forget that

thanksgiving is also distinctly commanded; we must praise God for His dealings with us, even though we cannot make them out at times. Let us see to it that the blessing we have gained is not temporary only, but that this wonderful peace may be with us always.

"God is teaching you in all these matters, and though our lessons are often hard to take to heart, yet we do get a delightfully close realization of His presence, in a way that we could not otherwise do. Pray God to make you cease from anxiety about yourself and your plans; just be willing to do the work our dear Father gives you at the time. I know from my own experience rest is found for the weary and the heavy laden, and a fulness of joy such as we can obtain in no other way. But I trust you are drinking from the Fountain Head already. My position has come to this, Am I living near my Saviour : then I am as happy as the day is long, and as light-hearted as a child. It may be that I have plenty of annoyances, but they don't trouble me when His presence is with me. Am I downcast and worried : then I am away from God. I have grieved the Holy Spirit by my sin. While this is my condition I am, thank God, in perfect health. When the body is sick the heart is no doubt often sad, and prone to be low-spirited by the very influence of the body over the mind. Yet to faith we know many of God's people have owed great peace in the midst of pain and severe illness."

At a later date he writes to the same friend :—

" I do trust you continue to find joy and rest in God. I am afraid my last letter to you was not a helpful one. Lesson : Never write to your friends when you are worried and anxious. In the first place, worry is absolutely wrong in a believer. Do you know this in the Psalms (cxix. 165)?—' Great peace have they which love Thy law,' and in Psalm lxviii. 19, new version, ' Blessed be the Lord, who daily beareth our burden.' Is not the latter a great improvement on the old version ?—' Daily loadeth us with benefits.' This was very precious, but not nearly so delightful as the new. I hope you are keeping quite well and strong in every respect this summer. Don't be unwise enough to think that we are serving God best by constant activity at the cost of head-aches and broken rest. I am getting to be of the opinion that we may be doing too much. We want— at least this is my own want—a higher quality of work. ' He that is entered into his rest, he also hath ceased from his own works, as God did from His ' (Heb. iv. 10). ' Let us labour therefore to enter into that rest' (ver. 11). Our labour should be to maintain unbroken communion with our blessed Lord ; then we shall have entire rest, and God abiding in us ; that which we do will not be ours, but His.

" I have not time for much reading now ; in fact, I am getting confined to a very small circle of litera-ture, of which the principal book is ' The Book.' "

Speaking of the Spirit's work among the medical students and in the hospital wards, he writes :—

" It is very delightful to see growth around you especially spiritual growth. It is worth suffering much (though I have no cause to talk of suffering, my joy has been so full), and coming a long way, to see Chinamen drinking in the living water."

Writing to the same friend, he notes down some comparisons between life in Nazareth and in China.

" Have you ever tried to picture what sort of a life our Lord led in Nazareth? Thompson, in his 'Land and the Book,' gives us some idea of what it must have been. The carpenters' tools of the present day in Judea are very similar to those used by the Chinese carpenter. The house, probably built of stone, must have been very bare and cheerless, especially among the poor with whom our Lord lived. Poverty and dirt generally go together, particularly in an Eastern climate. I wonder if the peasant of Nazareth was much cleaner or more comfortable than the Chinese peasant of the present day? They evidently had few belongings, for they could change their quarters without much hindrance from impedimenta. The villagers were unlettered and ignorant men ; they must have been chiefly occupied, as are the poor amongst the Chinese, in striving after the necessaries of life, in discussing ways and means. Christianity has, for thousands in our native land, converted earth into a paradise, compared with such a scene as this. To us the life of a Chinese peasant would be a perpetual martyrdom.

" ' Christ Jesus, who thought it not robbery to be

equal with God : but made Himself of no reputation, and took upon Him the form of a servant, and was made in the likeness of men.' From trying to picture, however imperfectly, something of our Lord's surroundings when on earth, I get new light upon the verse just quoted. What a constant martyrdom our Lord was ever going through while upon earth. Yet these external things were as nothing compared with the moral obliquity and spiritual deadness Jesus was always meeting with. How His pure heart must have been pained every day. Yet He was sustained by the constant peace of communion with the Father. Thank God we have the like blessed privilege open to us. 'Draw nigh to God, and He will draw nigh to you ; resist the devil, and he will flee from you.'"

On March 25th, 1887, he writes to his father :—

"Tien-tsin is very busy this year ; trade must be improving, judging by the large number of new arrivals in this settlement. It seems certain, too, that railways are to be introduced, at least in a small way. This the first step is the most important one, for if once started and accepted, their extension is only a matter of time. Marquis Tseng has the credit of finally convincing the Empress. He is stated to have said to Her Majesty, 'I have lived for ten years in Western lands, and have seen with my own eyes, and can bear personal testimony, that railways can only benefit our country and people, and cannot be harmful.' A small line is therefore sanctioned to connect some coal mines with Taku and Tien-tsin."

But while signs of progress were apparent, looking in the direction of a more complete opening up of the country, at the same time there were still signs, even in Tien-tsin, of that distrust and suspicion of foreigners which is constantly cropping up, and at this time it was to some extent directed against one who was generally acknowledged to be a public benefactor, *i.e.*, Dr. Mackenzie himself.

"There are a lot of unfortunate stories about kidnapping filling the air in Tien-tsin," he writes to a friend in China. "Some six or eight people have been seized and thrown into the yamen for stealing children, and it is said that they call themselves Roman Catholics, and profess to be in foreign employ. A scandalous paper was pasted in front of the bookshop vilifying the name of Jesus.

"Our English Consul called upon me to ask me to let him know what I should hear from the Chinese about the excitement. The French gunboat, after receiving orders to leave, has been stopped by order of the French Minister. I suppose the excitement will subside in a short while, but it is strange how these foolish reports are taken up and evidently believed.

"Mr. —— called in the other day to warn me that two different Chinese had told him that I was mixed up in the affair. The French Consul was supposed to have instigated the kidnapping, and I had supplied the medicines with which the children are supposed to be stupefied!"

The matter is thus referred to in the *Chinese Times* of that date : " For some time past the Chinese in and about Tien-tsin have been filled with consternation on account of the frequent occurrence of the kidnapping of children. Children disappeared, and the offenders could not be discovered."

It goes on to relate how five men were arrested, and after examination acknowledged their guilt, one of them declaring he had been bribed by the French missionaries to commit the crime.

" This statement, though suppressed by the magistrate, soon spread like wildfire through the city, and the story was embellished as it spread from mouth to mouth. The most absurd fables were invented : the children's bodies were used in the composition of foreign medicines ; their eyes were made into photographic chemicals ; they were sold to the steamers, etc., etc. On Friday evening last a popular rising against the foreign community of Tien-tsin seemed imminent. The Viceroy Li, who is absent in Peking, was communicated with, and immediately sent down most stringent orders to the Tien-tsin authorities to deal summarily with any persons attempting to make a disturbance, and to take prompt measures to restore tranquillity. The state of affairs during Friday, Saturday, and Sunday was critical, but the precautions taken by the authorities have now removed all danger of an outbreak. A body of Chinese troops was guarding the settlement on Saturday and Sunday nights."

In a letter to his brother, written at this time, Dr. Mackenzie says :—

" It is a great blessing when one can cast care to the winds, and acquire perfect freedom from anxiety. This is evidently much easier for some than others ; one thing I feel sure of, it is not hard work that kills, but worry. I think I am very little troubled in this way now, thank God ; for instance, I have fifty-four in-patients under my charge just now, nearly all surgical cases and of the greatest anxiety, and yet I am not in the least worried, though my time is very fully occupied."

Later on he writes to his father :—

" We badly need another medical missionary for Tien-tsin, and in November last I wrote, offering to pay passage money and to guarantee salary, if only the Directors would find a man, but up to the present we have heard nothing. It is my private opinion that our Society is hardly in touch with the best kind of men in England. The latitudinarianism of so many Congregational ministers in England is a death-blow to the missionary spirit of our Churches. Look at our Society, heavily in debt, and hundreds of the members of Congregational Churches giving annual subscriptions of one or two guineas who have incomes of some thousands a year, and yet will not increase their subscriptions. What more forcible evidence is wanted of their lack of faith in missions ? "

Doubtless, had Dr. Mackenzie lived he would have modified these statements ; but he had been strongly impressed and pained, during his visit home, by the small interest generally felt in foreign missions.

"As to the success of our work, I think it has been wonderful, especially considering our unfitness for the great struggle with darkness and sin in this land. Were we and the Churches who send us full of the Spirit of God, and sufficiently humbled and emptied of self for our Heavenly Father to manifest His marvellous power in and through us, of course success would be vastly more. But considering, as I say, what we are and what the Churches at home are, the results of our labour have been such as to call forth praise and thanksgiving to God. The work here is manifestly God's, and none but His. I have men around me in the hospital and medical school who are so clearly born of God that there can be no question about it. The great sin of the present day is emphatically unbelief. That is, unbelief in God, for there is plenty of faith to be found, only unfortunately it is not the right kind of faith ; it is faith in self, faith in *our* institutions, in *our* schemes, in our own wisdom. Faith in our Lord Jesus must ever go hand in hand with deep humility, as in the case of the centurion, and true humility, I fancy, is very scarce in the present day. Excuse my rambling on, and please do not think me downhearted about my work. I am full of hope, for never have I spent what I trust has been such a profitable year during my short life. The openings I have here are more than I could ever have expected. The Viceroy is remarkably kind to me, and thoughtful of my work. There is plenty of money and abundance of opportunities, and the work could be extended indefinitely if we only had more men of the right stamp."

In June of the same year the Doctor writes to his father :—

"It is a great privilege to serve the Lord here in China. I feel so thankful to God for giving me this honour, and for leading me into a deeper appreciation of it. In our hospital work we are daily meeting with men who have never heard of the way of salvation, and who have no joy in life, and it is our delightful privilege to tell them of a Saviour mighty to save. But, oh! we need power ; the deadness of these souls is something awful ; their utter ignorance of what sin is, the fearful lethargy into which they have fallen, all reveal that our one great essential is power,--Divine, life-giving power. And bless God we have all this in Christ. When at the creation all was darkness and chaos, it was He who said, ' Let there be light, and there was light.' And it was He too who breathed into man's nostrils the breath of life, and man ' became a living soul.' If we did not constantly bear this in mind we should get disheartened, or else faithless in view of what we meet with daily. But not only have we to look back into the past for evidences of His mighty power : He vouchsafes to manifest it even here and now, to cheer our faith and to encourage to renewed energy. It is our joy to see from among these lifeless souls men truly born again, and exemplifying the spiritual life clearly and brightly amongst their fellows. It is a wonderful sight thus to see a dead soul come to life again ; no wonder there is joy in heaven. The Lord has been so gracious to me of late, giving me so much joy in my life, so much thorough satisfaction and rest. I can truly bless His holy Name for all His wonderful goodness and mercy towards me. Outward circumstances have very little to do with heart peace or real heart satisfaction. It is the presence of the living Saviour, and this alone, in our lives which gives it.

" I am so glad to hear you are keeping so well, dear father. I hope you get little Maggie to learn some sweet hymns, and sing them to you. I should so like to hear that she sings praise to her loving Father in heaven. Do you often talk to her about how Jesus loves her ? I think it is a mistake to think that children do not or cannot enter into the comprehension of spiritual things."

Writing to his friend Colonel Duncan, with whom Mackenzie had corresponded at as frequent intervals as his busy life would permit ever since he came to China, he says :—

" Oh, why do not more of the Lord's people come to this land ? It is evident that He is wanting to pour out salvation upon the people of China, but is hindered by the lack of messengers. I have just come from a meeting we hold every Friday evening for the study of the Scriptures, a believers' meeting ;

and it was indeed a hallowed time, for the Lord's presence was there in large measure. It is for the special help of the dispensers and ward-attendants, who are all Christians, and the converted patients join in. As one after another spoke as the Lord moved him, I could not help blessing God for the manifestation of His power. Only a few years ago many of these men were heathen, worshipping idols, and now they know God, and enjoy communion with Him. All are working Christians, seeking daily to teach and lead into the light the patients who throng our wards ; and the Lord has given us such access to the people, for from hundreds of miles they come seeking healing, and place themselves with childlike confidence in our hands.

" As to myself, the dear Lord is blessing me beyond measure. I cannot recount His goodness, the instances are too numerous even to mention ; I can only praise and extol His holy Name. Since my return to China I have led, humanly speaking, a very lonely life, but the Saviour has led me in a way I could not have imagined. These last three years have been full of instruction to me. Though one of the Lord's chosen people, I was previously so ignorant of Him ; now, through His great mercy, I have been learning what it is in some measure to walk with Him and to hold close communion with Him. Oh, He has been so good to me in filling up my life with such unutterable joy and peace.

" I have been greatly blessed in being kept from

anxiety. 'In nothing be anxious,' etc., has proved
of great comfort to me, both in regard to my
family sorrows and my hospital cares, for with so
many patients, and most of them surgical operation
cases often of the greatest severity, humanly speaking
I could scarcely have borne the strain; yet I think I
was never in better health, and my heart as light and
free from care as I could wish. Excuse my writing
so much about myself, but I would testify to the
wondrous grace and mercy of the Lord, whose I
am."

CHAPTER XV.

GROWING IN GRACE.

CHAPTER XV.

GROWING IN GRACE.

THE Christian life was always spoken of by St. Paul as a progressive thing, the high aim placed before every believer being that of attaining to the measure of the stature of the fulness of Christ. And as God, through His servant, would never have called His people to tasks they could not perform, to heights impossible of attainment, we know that the Father of our Lord Jesus Christ has pledged Himself to supply all that is necessary to effect in us that to which He calls us.

In Dr. Mackenzie's life this principle of growth was strikingly manifest. He had always been an earnest and devoted missionary since first he set foot on Chinese soil, and he had ever given great prominence to the evangelistic side of Medical Mission work.

But during the last year or so of his life his growth in likeness to His Divine Master was evident to all, and that passion for souls which can only possess any heart as the result of the indwelling of God's Holy Spirit in abundant measure, became the inspiring thought of his life. During his early years in Tien-tsin

319

he had, to some slight extent, shared in the innocent and healthful recreations of his fellow-countrymen in the community. He was fond of riding, and, as we have seen, experienced great benefit from his morning gallop over the plains; he enjoyed skating, and during the long northern winter used to secure almost daily a limited time for this healthful recreation, while during the rest of the year he not unfrequently took a turn at lawn tennis. Some will perhaps look upon it as a defect in his Christian character, that as time went on he began to feel such an absorbing interest in the things that are unseen and eternal, that Bible study filled up most of his leisure time, when his manifold professional duties were finished, almost to the exclusion of ordinary social intercourse.

He rarely took any recreation, with the exception of his daily " constitutional," which he looked upon in the light of a duty for health's sake. He used to say sometimes, that on account of those in our Eastern communities who frequently complain of the absence of most missionaries from all their entertainments and seasons of recreation, he had determined to make a fair trial, and see as much of English society as time would allow ; but he had not found this experiment a success, and had therefore given it up.

Without doubt the highest ideal of the Christian life is that a believer in Jesus, following closely in the footsteps of his Divine Master, should be able to go into all society, as Christ Himself did, shedding around him the blessed influence of a life filled with the spirit of love and boundless charity ; for Christians are to be in the world as their Master was in it, to bless, and comfort, and strengthen. This is the ideal life, but it is perhaps only attained by the few.

It is no unfrequent circumstance to see the Christian, who has earnestly desired to be " in the world, yet not of it," by slow degrees losing the freshness of his first love, and finding, by sad experience, how difficult a task it is to keep his garments unspotted from the world. To escape this trying ordeal, the monks and hermits of old separated themselves entirely from the world of daily life and business, shunning the holy and happy influences of the home life which our Saviour Himself had blessed and sanctified.

We think they were wrong now, those holy men of old, though we honour their noble lives and utter self-abnegation, and we remember at the same time that our Lord's life was not of the ascetic type at all. He never shrank from any festive gathering to which He was invited, and was found mixing with every grade of society that Judea had to offer. Yet He ever went, like the physician into the plague-stricken district, to heal and to save.

So that in these matters it is not for us to judge each other, but for each to seek guidance as special circumstances arise, remembering that, as one has well said, both as regards the saints of ancient times and the followers of Christ in these later days, " God will judge us at last by our sincerity, and not by our wisdom."

Dr. Mackenzie was, however, well known in the Tien-tsin community in his professional capacity, for he was frequently called in for consultation by Drs. Frazer and Irwin ; and as one among them wrote, when he was called away, " He had endeared himself greatly by his kindness and singular delicacy of manner, while his skill as a physician inspired universal confidence."

In a letter to his father during the summer he says :—

" I have not written lately, I have been altogether too busy. Dr. Irwin, the only doctor at present in the settlement, was taken ill with acute dysentery, and I had to attend him and his patients. He is better, and is now gone to Taku for the sea-air, and I have still to look after his practice. The foreign community numbers over three hundred, and this month of June we are having extra hot weather, temperature over 100° Fahr. in the shade, and so more people get sick. I am happily very well, but work has too much of a rush about it just now to please me. Dr. Macfarlane is helping me now with the students, so that frees me somewhat."

Dr. Mackenzie always felt a great admiration and sympathy for men of noble character with whom he came in contact, who were hindered by " honest doubt " from any open profession of faith in Christ or an active Christian life. " They are not far from the kingdom," he would say sometimes.

At his death a slip of paper was found within the

covers of his Bible, on which subjects for prayer for each day of the week were noted down. Among more general subjects, he had particular days for prayer for friends in England, for the medical students, and for certain members of the foreign community in whom he felt specially interested.

His fondness for Bible study has been alluded to. A striking evidence of this was found in the Bible he had in use at the time of his death, which bore the date of January 1888, and could therefore have only been in use for about three months. Passages had been marked in almost every part of both Old and New Testaments ; while whole books, such as Exodus and the Song of Songs, had been carefully studied, and the lives of particular prophets and kings, like Samuel and Hezekiah, had been closely followed, many appropriate and thoughtful remarks being noted down in the margin.

His own circumstances formed the key to many of the passages marked. "As a man chasteneth his son so the Lord thy God chasteneth thee" (Deut. viii. 5 "Why art thou cast down, O my soul ? and why art thou disquieted within me ? Hope thou in God : for I shall yet praise Him who is the health of my countenance " (Psalm xliii. 5). Against the passage in Deut. viii. 17, " My power and the might of mine hand hath gotten me this wealth," occurs the word " Blind ! " probably suggested by an undercurrent of thought regarding the great facilities and large pecuniary help God had granted him for carrying on the hospital, together with the accumulated savings which had provided a large reserve fund for the future carrying on of the medical work, as he hoped.

Ezekiel's call and commission had been carefully studied, and also the life of King Hezekiah, the last passage marked being, singularly enough, " And all Judah and the inhabitants of Jerusalem did him honour at his death ; " a statement which could be used with equal appropriateness to describe the state of feeling in the city in which Dr. Mackenzie lived, when so shortly after he was removed by death.

A few months before, a friend had sent out to the Doctor a copy of the well-known text-book " Daily Light on the Daily Path." He had found this so helpful, that it was his intention to translate and arrange it for the benefit of the Chinese converts, had his life been spared.*

Dr. Mackenzie had always a strong conviction that the Christian life should be one of gladness and rejoicing, and that we have no right to allow the sorrows and trials which may shadow our path to destroy our peace, or fill our hearts with undue care. Speaking one day of a person who was suffering severely from depression, and whose convalescence from a severe illness had thus been hindered, he remarked :—

" Yes, I am well aware he has enough to trouble him, but then we have no right to dwell morbidly

---

* This work has been undertaken by two members of the London Mission, Miss Moreton and the Rev. Hopkyn Rees.

upon the trials of this life. If I allowed myself to dwell upon my own sorrows I might be the most sorrowful of men, but this is not God's will in sending us these means of discipline. We are rather to rise above them, and find our joy in work for Him."

Dr. Mackenzie was always deeply interested in the welfare of the seamen of the various ships of war which wintered in Tien-tsin, and was a supporter of the Gospel Temperance Movement. He had little faith, however, in any but spiritual methods as a means of helping and elevating them. Indeed, his one idea in all his intercourse with his fellow-men was to bring them into personal contact with a living Saviour.

The Doctor almost invariably received great assistance from the naval surgeons of the various nationalities, and formed a warm and lasting friendship with some of them. Of one he writes :—

"On Wednesday afternoons we give a holiday to the medical students, and then I try and get a walk with Dr. ——, a very dear Christian friend on board the English gunboat. When you do meet with a Christian officer in the navy you find him an aggressive one, a sort of Hedley Vicars. It may seem strange to you to hear there are so few Christian men out here, and it is strange ; but whether or not it is the result of Eastern life, with its greater luxury and ease for foreigners, it is a fact that, with few exceptions, the religious life is discarded in China by our fellow-countrymen. Such a statement as this would be badly received by many, for great numbers claim to be Christians; but what men object to is 'being religious,' as they like to call it; in other words, trying to follow Christ."

Referring to the Memoir of his friend, John Gordon of Pitburg and Parkhill, which he had lately been reading, the Doctor says :—

"His was a noble life; such singleness of purpose and consecration is only, alas, too rare. So many of us fear to be singular, and fear what men will think of us, rather than simply what our Master would have us do. I lent the book to a friend of mine, a bright young Christian, who stands almost alone among his fellows in witnessing for the truth. One does admire a man who takes up his cross and follows Christ in these communities in China, for it is a real cross-bearing."

In a letter to a friend, a former Tien-tsin resident, he says :—

"I trust you will be settled in a port where you will have happy service for the Lord. This has been an unusually worldly winter, even for Tien-tsin. They have had the municipal band playing at the skating rink on Sundays regularly. The introduction of so many French and German residents has tended to turn our Sunday into one after the continental model,—games and paper hunts and other amusements being held more frequently, I think, on Sunday than on other days, and printed notices to this effect come round in the most open manner. Well, perhaps this is not a thing to be altogether sorry for, as it compels the Lord's children to separate themselves more thoroughly from the world."

Dr. Mackenzie longed earnestly to see the gospel making rapid progress in China, and for this reason always warmly welcomed the arrival of new missionaries.

In the autumn of 1887 he was cheered by the coming of some whose arrival was a source of special satisfaction to him. The first of these was one with whom he had been engaged in Christian work in Bristol many years before, and whose way had been opened up, after many days, to come out to the mission field in connection with the China Inland Mission. His letter to this friend of former days contains the following passage :—

" Let me give you a hearty welcome to this land in which I have lived now for twelve years, and certainly bless the Lord for giving me the honour and privilege of ever coming here."

The other missionary in whose arrival he took a special interest was the medical colleague who came out to join his friend Mr. Gilmour in the Mongolian Mission.

More than eighteen months before, Dr. Mackenzie had been appointed by the Tien-tsin Committee, on account of his deep interest in the matter, to write an urgent appeal to the Directors of the L. M. S. for a medical colleague for Mr. Gilmour in Mongolia ; and so deeply did he feel the necessity of such an appointment, that after pleading the fact that our Lord avoided sending forth His disciples singly, since He knew how dependent we are upon human sympathy, he went on to say, that even, if necessary, he was willing that his fondly-cherished scheme of having a second medical missionary for his colleague in Tien-tsin should, for the time, be set aside, and the next doctor sent to North China be designated to the Mongolian Mission.

It was therefore a matter of special rejoicing to Dr. Mackenzie when, after long waiting, the news came that a medical colleague for Mr. Gilmour was on the way; and he wrote the following letter of welcome to Dr. Roberts, who, in the providence of God, was destined, in the short space of a few months, to take up and carry on Dr. Mackenzie's own work, when he received his sudden summons to the higher service above.

" Allow me to offer you a most loving welcome to China. I think this is, beyond other countries, the field for Medical Missions. The work is a glorious one, and I thank God that I have been honoured to take some part in the effort to bring China to Christ. I am sure you too will bless the day that first brought you to this land."

After an appreciative reference to his valued friend and Dr. Roberts' contemplated colleague, Mr. Gilmour, the Doctor concludes the letter with the following texts : " My soul, wait thou *only* upon God ; for my expectation is from Him. He only is my rock : I shall not be moved. Power belongeth unto God " (Psalm lxii.).

It was decided that Dr. Roberts should remain in Tien-tsin for some months, to get a start with the language. They shared the same house together, and, as is evident from Dr. Mackenzie's constant reference to his new friend in his home letters, this arrangement was a source of much satisfaction to him.

" I am very well, and the work is prospering," he writes. " It is such a pleasure to have a congenial friend in the same house with one. . . . I think it is good for digestion, not to speak of other benefits— one eats food with more enjoyment. We have such pleasant walks and talks together. Dr. Roberts is well acquainted with Mr. Meyer of Leicester, who is doing such good service for the Church of Christ."

Dr. Mackenzie held strongly to the doctrines of grace, and had no sympathy at all with the new theology.

" What do you think of Spurgeon's action ? " he asks in a letter to his father. " I am delighted with the stand he has taken, and trust it may do much to awaken thoughtful students of the Bible to the danger of many of the theories floating around. If only it leads men to test for themselves—to search and prove whether these things be so—it will be doing good service. We are too much inclined to take things at second hand. Now that we have a good revised Bible no one need say, ' I cannot go to the fountain head for information.' "

The presence of two medical colleagues in Tien-tsin at this time made it possible for Dr. Mackenzie to carry out his long-cherished purpose of paying a visit to the country districts around Tien-tsin, with the view of strengthening the many scattered Christians who had been led to a knowledge of Jesus as their Saviour within the wards of the hospital. Many of them had received baptism upon a profession of their faith in Christ, and had returned to their homes to witness for Him in places where the gospel had never before been heard.

And it was thus that he spent the last Christmas and New Year's holidays of his life, in the company of one of his dispensers, who, like all his assistants and servants, was his devoted friend. During this three weeks of itineration he lived with the country people as a guest in their homes, sharing their humble hospitality, and endearing himself to them in a way that will not soon be forgotten.

It was Dr. Mackenzie's intention to write an account of this journey, which was to him a source of much encouragement and rejoicing, because it enabled him to see how widely the Lord was using the work done in the hospital wards, and the men there brought to a knowledge of the Saviour, to spread the good news of salvation far and wide through the surrounding districts. The discomforts of such a journey in the bitter cold of a North China winter, the separation from friends at the New Year's season of reunion, were of small account to him in comparison with the joy he had in seeing the progress of God's kingdom in the land, and finding the men who had confessed Christ in Tien-tsin standing firm amid the trials and persecution of their own home life.

From various sources, such as note-books, letters, etc., I glean the following account of this last journey of itineration :—

" The patients who have given hopeful evidence of a change of heart, under the teaching of the Spirit of God, often live three or four or more days' journey from Tien-tsin, and except in the event of their visiting us again, we have few opportunities of following them up. I took advantage of the valued presence of Drs. Macfarlane and Roberts to take a several weeks' trip into the country at the end of the year, for the purpose of visiting the homes of some of my old patients, to see how their Christianity was wearing among their neighbours. I had a companion in one of the dispensers, Chang Kung Mao, and a very encouraging journey it proved.

" In making such a trip one has to hire a cart, without springs of course, and two mules to draw the vehicle, into which you put your bedding and such articles as you deem necessary for the journey. I was well wrapped up, having a sheep-skin coat, dog-skin stockings, felt boots, and felt and fur cap. The Chinese have no fires, except for cooking, and do not depend upon artificial heat, but upon a super-abundance of clothing, to keep the body warm.

"On the first day we journeyed over a barren plain, mostly following the course of the Grand Canal. The land had been under water through the canal having broken its banks, and there was much distress and poverty in the district. We stayed the first night at Ning-hai-hien, and spoke to three of the men belonging to the inn about Jesus ; one, an old man of seventy, seemed much interested. The best inns have brick beds called kangs, but most of them off the high road have only a raised earthen platform at one end of the room, which serves both for bed and seat. The windows in every case are made of paper, and are of course full of holes ; the floor is of earth, and altogether inns in China are not desirable places. But one soon gets used to anything, and if your health holds good all goes well. Being very hungry from the cold, dry air circulating around all day, when you get in at night you get some hot food, in rare cases rice and a little meat, and after your meal you feel inclined to go to sleep. Your surroundings are too uncomfortable to want dwelling upon, so you pull your cap over your ears, dispense with your boots, the only article of attire you remove, and throwing yourself on the mattress, cover yourself with the native bed-quilt, and go to sleep.

"The second morning we rose two or three hours before the sun, and soon after ate half a hot sweet potato, weighing a catty. We had rather a tiresome time before reaching the next town. The carter came to a part of the road where there was ice, and insisted upon trying to cross, even though it looked unsafe. We urged him to return, but he only beat the mules the more, and first one and then the other floundered into the water, breaking the ice in their struggles. The left cart wheel went through the ice into a hole, and we were all but over. Finally the shaft mule fell down, and had to be unharnessed, and then the carter agreed to turn back. He harnessed first one mule and then the other to the back of the cart, but it would not move; the man was meanwhile cursing the mules with all his might, calling them by every opprobrious name, though it was solely due to his own obstinacy that this trouble had come. Some passing carters were appealed to for help, but they paid no heed; at last some poor travellers on foot came along, and they helped, with the mules, to drag the cart out of the ice.

"The next day we dined at a place where a fair was being held. All sorts of things were offered for sale on extempore stalls in the very midst of the streets. It looked like a picture of Vanity Fair in the ' Pilgrim's Progress.' Every imaginable Chinese requirement was there, from horses and bullocks to coloured cloths, drapery, and eatables.

"We have great difficulty in finding our way on this barren plain, for the roads are constantly cross-ing and dividing. Nor were our difficulties over when we had succeeded in our search, and reached the village or market-town we were seeking.

"As an example, let me describe what took place

at a village called Ba-wang. Upon entering we soon
found ourselves surrounded by a curious crowd, eager
to gaze at the strange spectacle of a foreigner in the
place. Not seeing the face of the friend we are
seeking among them, we enquire of the nearest person,
' Will you kindly direct us to the house of Mr. Chang ? '
' He does not live here,' is the immediate reply,
uttered most emphatically, as though to shut off at
once all hope. ' But isn't this village called Ba-wang ? '
' Yes, it is.' ' Well, then, we know that Mr. Chang does
live here.' ' Oh, it's that man, is it ? ' as if waking up
suddenly to lively recollection. ' Well, he has gone
from home ; he does not live in this place now.
There is no man of that name here at all ! '

"These are evidently impromptu answers, given
without thought, so we have to begin and make more
particular enquiries, and give some explanations.
' Look here, friends,' we say, 'we know Mr. Chang ;
he was a patient in the Tien-tsin hospital ; he had
bad eyes for over four years, one was nearly blind.
He is about so tall, is a thin man, and has three
children ; now, you see, we are acquainted with him.
We are on the road travelling, and have called to pay
him a visit. Now won't you tell us where he lives ?
Really now, we have not come to collect a debt, nor
do we want to borrow travelling expenses from him ! '

"These remarks are rendered necessary on account
of the suspiciousness of the villagers, who have a great
antipathy to strangers, and evidently look upon a man
as an enemy till he has proved himself to be a friend

'We assure you we have only come to see him. We are Christians.' By-and-bye the suspicions begin to disappear.

"'What did you say his name was?' they enquire. 'Chang? No, there is no one of that name.' Suddenly some one in the crowd exclaims, 'Why, it's "G'ar"!' calling the man by some pet or nickname he has borne since childhood. Apparently in many cases their own proper names are not used or even known among the villagers. 'Oh, if it's that man you mean, G'ar lives at the other end of the village.' And so at last we are allowed to discover our friend's whereabouts, and receive a warm welcome from him.

"At another large market-town, where the Roman Catholics were strong, we sought two men of the name of Hu, who had formerly been patients; but amongst a large clan of the same name we could not trace our friends. At another place we found a Roman Catholic church, built with brick, after a foreign model, with little turrets and a large crucifix on the top. There was a foreign priest living there, so I called on him, and he kindly took me over the church. He spoke no English, and had lived in this village of two hundred families for three years. He said there were thirty families of converts, and they had built the church at their own cost. The interior was rather dirty, and the pictures of the Virgin and the saints were rather tawdry.

"We next made our way to Hsiao-shih, where four

men lived who had been baptized, all bearing the same surname, Hu. Kung Mao, the dispenser, went on to seek them out, leaving me in the cart. He found all our friends were absent at a large fair in the neighbourhood, but as soon as their relatives heard who we were, they came out and seized hold of us, and literally took possession. They would not hear of our going to put up at the inn. Leading the mules to the door of the father of one of the ex-patients, they quickly conveyed all our belongings on to the kang of an inner room.

"After a while the son returned from the fair, and gave us a hearty welcome. He is a fine young fellow of twenty-two, the eldest son of a rich farmer, who farms his own land of one hundred and fifty Chinese acres. He reads well, is intelligent, and was baptized while in the hospital; he was an in-patient, suffering from rheumatism. His father is a thoughtful, intelligent man of over forty, who treated us in the most hospitable manner, insisting upon feeding our carters and attending to our mules. He pressed us to remain with him some days. Though not professedly a Christian, he has learned a good deal of the doctrine from his son.

"We were in the houses of three other Christians, and saw not a trace of idolatry anywhere.

"Another man, the son of a well-to-do shopkeeper, had been a patient; he reads well, and keeps his father's accounts in the shop. He has an elder brother, who seemed bright and interested, but cannot read. We dined with this family, and afterwards preached in their house to many visitors.

"Two other old patients, each over forty years of age, lived in this place. One of them, before his conversion, was known as 'No. 2 Teacher.' He is not an educated man, but has a gift for story-telling. Before he came to Tien-tsin he did not know a character ; now he can read his Bible. We dined at his house and preached there, Kung Mao telling with power the story of the prodigal son to the assembled villagers. This man is poor, and his eyes still give him trouble ; he has no land, but works for others ; he has a son in business in the place. Another man, named Shen, is less earnest ; he wished us, however, to go and dine with him the day we left. He farms his own land of forty acres. He was in the hospital for granular lids, and improved under treatment, but the trouble has recurred. These four Christians meet together for conversation about the Word of God and prayer, the three earnest ones every evening. Deng-Yung joins them occasionally, but it is not convenient for him, on account of his bad eyesight, to go regularly at night. Tao-ping's father told us that after the Chinese New Year he should give them a room to hold worship in,—an old schoolroom, which is at present let. The interest in this village is great, and the Lord gave us an open door in every direction. The Shen family earnestly begged us to stay longer with them, but we rather hesitated at putting them to so much expense in entertaining us, as they would

22

allow us to pay for nothing, and every meal was a feast.

"Tao-ping, the son, rode over on his mule to the next town we wished to visit, to show us the way. The man we wished to see, a Christian named Wang, is poor, having only ten acres of land. He gave us a hearty welcome, and in the presence of a crowd of fellow-villagers testified for Christ. We spoke a few words to the people, left some books, exhorted Wang to keep near Jesus, and soon left. Wang's nephew, a young man of twenty, said he had learnt the doctrines from his uncle ; he believed in Christ, and was hoping, after the New Year, to come to Tien-tsin and receive baptism. A number of the villagers had learnt something of the truth from Wang.

"At the next place we sought for a man of the name of Ch'en, but found he was away from home at the district city, where he was a party in a lawsuit, which had been brought against him by another man, relating to his right of ownership in the shops where he carried on his business. We were disappointed at not seeing Ch'en, as he had been long in the hospital with lupus of the face. However, we laid the matter before the Lord, and prayed for guidance and for a blessing on the man, and went on to the inn. It was the worst we had come across yet, and after our snug quarters at the Shen village we felt the cold bitterly on this Christmas Eve. The walls were made of sun-dried mud bricks, unplastered,

and so the wind came through them as through a
sieve, and it was so bitterly cold that we did not get
much sleep.

"Morning was welcome, and by daylight we were
on our way. We considered whether we should go
to the city and seek for Ch'en ; but we thought the
search would prove so difficult, that we decided to go
on to the next patient on our list. On our way,
however, we most unexpectedly met Mr. Ch'en. He
had finished his business on the previous evening, and
hearing from a friend that some people from Tien-tsin
were seeking him, he started off first thing in the
morning to look for us at our inn. We had started
before he arrived, and had we gone by the other
road should have missed him. We felt we had been
guided of the Lord. We returned with Ch'en to his
home, and entered his father's house. The father, a
most courteous old gentleman of sixty-five, received
us most kindly, as did also his mother and younger
brother. The room was soon full of neighbours, to
whom we preached, and afterwards we all, Ch'en included, prayed together. We were hungry and tired,
and soon after went to our inn and had a late
breakfast. This was on Christmas Day. Ch'en's
father wished us to stay with them, but as they were
not well off we declined. After this we preached
until quite tired out, speaking on the parable of
the fig-tree, the prodigal son, the miracle of healing
the palsied man borne of four, and blind Bartimæus.
Ch'en did some preaching and teaching too, and told

us that his father and next neighbour were well inclined to the gospel; the former was very intelligent, and had read some of the New Testament. The innkeeper, who was a friend of Ch'en's, treated us most kindly; he knew something of the doctrine some time before, as Mr. Perkins had stayed at his inn and left some books.

"At the next town we sought for a man named Lin, about forty years of age, who had left the hospital nine months ago, after undergoing an operation for gangrene, having had his right foot removed. He was originally a very small farmer; after losing his foot he was unable to cultivate his land, so he had to sell it, and being, for a countryman, a very good scholar, his fellow-clansmen, all with the same surname, made him schoolmaster in the village, and on our arrival we found him installed in this capacity.

"But alas for his Christianity! No sooner had he reached home than he began to trouble himself as to how he would ever be able to maintain himself now he was a cripple. As it seemed as if he was entirely dependent upon the help of his neighbours, he was much afraid of offending them, so he kept silent about the doctrine, and concealed the fact that he was a Christian, and none of his neighbours knew it. As soon as we reached his house he began to explain to us why he had not preached to the villagers; he dare not offend them, as they sent their children to be taught by him. We preached for some time to the neighbours, who flocked into the schoolroom ; but they took little interest in what we said, we fear, because Lin had been hiding his light under a bushel.

" After exhorting Lin to cease to fear man and to fear God, and so get peace in his heart, we gave him some books and a calendar, and left. Next day we crossed the Grand Canal, and made our way to a place where two brothers named T'sai were living, who were farmers.

" They were in the hospital about ten months ago ; the younger brother's foot requiring amputation, the elder brother was there nursing him. There were five brothers in the family, and the elder was the only scholar among them ; that is to say, none of the others knew a character, while he could read and write well. He took from the first a deep interest in the gospel, and soon declared himself on the Lord's side. He was a most hopeful, earnest, and solid character, while his younger brother was dull and apathetic, and though he also desired baptism before leaving the hospital, I think it was without any deep conviction of sin, but rather at the instigation and under the teaching of his brother. The truth was very real to the elder man, and we hoped much from our visit to him.

" Kung Mao went on before to find the family out, and came back with the sad news that Djen Dsung was dead. The very day after he brought back his younger brother, recovered after the operation, he was himself taken ill, with what disease they could not tell us. They said that for over eight months he lay ill on his bed, and all the doctors within reach failed to relieve him, and he died just a month before our arrival. We went with the lame brother into the house and saw the old mother ; their father was still alive, but he was away at a fair.

"The old lady received us most kindly, and told us how her son had longed to see us before he died, and had wept because it was impossible,—wept several times, the poor mother said, and was always praying, reading his Bible, and talking to them about the doctrine. How strange it seems, humanly speaking, that this man should be called away just when he had such a work to do ; but God knows best.

"The younger brother seemed very listless, but the mother was quite hopeful, and sat with us all the time we were there, and from her evident interest we directed our remarks mainly to her. The father, it seems, is still an idolater.

"At another town we met three more Christians, and had a service with them at our inn. One of them, named Yang, had been at the hospital waiting on his son, who afterwards died. He was baptized before leaving ; he owns several shops, one a cash shop. He had lent his Bible to a friend, who had not returned it. The second, named Chang, is engaged as buyer in a large distillery. He buys grains and dates, and is constantly travelling about the country. All these three men can read well and pray aloud.

" At the next place we visited we stayed the night. Miau-chia-tswang is a town where idolatry is rife. When ill the people invite priests to come to their houses ; they burn incense and go through idolatrous ceremonies, but give no medicine. A Christian named Ch'en, whose house we were seeking, a good scholar who reads well, we found to be well known as a believer in the place. He has met with much opposition. One man had learned the doctrine from him, and believed in Christ, but feared to confess his faith on account of the displeasure of his friends. His father and mother knew something of the gospel, but were very indifferent. We preached to them and to many neighbours.

" At the last place we visited, about thirty miles from Tien-tsin, we saw a man named Leo, who had been in the hospital two years ago. He is a farmer, with one hundred acres of land, and also a salt merchant, scraping the salt off the surface of the soil, and afterwards putting it through some process to purify it. He has two children, ten and eleven years of age ; the elder had committed the catechism to memory. He has also two brothers ; one of them is an educated man and keeps a school. Our old patient only possessed the catechism and a tract on the parable of the prodigal son. He is a good scholar, speaks well, and is fond of preaching the doctrine. The keeper of our inn is a friend of his, and seems a most hopeful man."

CHAPTER XVI.

LAST THINGS.

CHAPTER XVI.

LAST THINGS.

THE Chinese New Year's season is the great holiday time of the whole year in the Middle Kingdom ; even the poorest coolies try to take their ease for a few days, and almost all business is suspended for nearly a fortnight. So that for a few days the necessaries of life are purchased with difficulty.

Of course every one is too busily engaged in anticipations of pleasure-making to attend to any bodily ailments, and at this season the dispensaries and hospitals are almost deserted.

Consequently Dr. Mackenzie was able to take a hard-earned holiday, which, as we find from his diary, he spent in answering an accumulation of correspondence with friends both in England and China.

" Chinese New Year is the great occasion for paying off old debts," he writes, " and I am following the very good custom set by the Chinese in this respect, in trying to wipe off some epistolary debts."

To his friend Dr. Atterbury of Peking he wrote as follows :—

" I wish more would write for the Journal *(The*

347

China Medical Missionary Journal), and send a variety, not merely confining themselves to medical matters. *There is the missionary side of the question.*

" Praise the Lord we have had a good year here in the hospital. Thirty-nine patients were baptized during the year. I feel so grateful to the Lord for thus working, when there is so much in me that is displeasing to Him. Yet all the more is the glory His.

" He is teaching me some things ; one to have more child-like faith, to believe that what He says He means. And when Jesus says, ' Ask, and ye shall receive,' I now know, as I never before did, that Jesus will answer my prayers, perhaps sometimes by not giving me that for which I pray. This year, God helping me, I intend to trust Him more to use the hospital to the salvation of souls. I was searching out all the promises concerning prayer in the Word the other day. Oh, they are so full and wonderful ; I am so shamefaced that I have been so dumb before the Lord for so long. Then, as to united prayer, two of you agreeing together : we have had a united noon-day prayer-meeting, just a few of us, which has been much blessed to myself.

" Simplicity, directness, straightforwardness—these are all needed in prayer. I have been for years hypocritically repeating words in prayer, when I never expected God to answer. How displeasing to a loving Father is such conduct. The Lord forgive me and teach me ! Isn't it a privilege to trust the Saviour ? "

To Mr. Stooke, of the China Inland Mission,
Chefoo, with whom he had been engaged in Christian
work many years before in Bristol, he writes :—

" I suppose you are hard at work at this delightful
language. Well, it only wants pegging away at, and
patience wins.

" I was away in the country on a journey last
December, a thing I cannot often manage, but I
have two medical colleagues for this winter, Drs.
Macfarlane and Roberts. I had a good time, and
was prospered by the good Lord. Then when I got
back we had a capital week of prayer. Gilmour was
in from Mongolia, and we managed to get two little
Bible readings every day, and God blessed us."

During this New Year season Dr. Mackenzie also
wrote the following interesting report of the work
done in the hospital wards and dispensary during
the year :—

" In accordance with the wishes of the Directors, I beg to
forward the following report of the work in my hands for
1887 :—

" *Tien-tsin Medical Mission.*

" *Dispensary.*—Number of attendances during the year,
13,799.

" *Hospital.*—Number of in-patients during the year, 591.

" *Medical School.*—Number of students in training, 9.

" The in-patients were thirty-five more than during the
year 1886, and I think they were drawn from a better class
in the social scale. The work in all its branches has gone
on uninterruptedly. The presence and help of my dear
friends, Drs. Macfarlane and Roberts, have been of great

assistance to the cause, and a source of much comfort to myself. While naturally their main energies are directed to the study of the language, yet they have found time to render valuable help—not the least valuable being their earnest daily prayer for God's blessing. Dr. Macfarlane has also given much service in the instruction of the medical students, thus freeing me for more direct Christian labour amongst the patients.

" In its medical aspect the work has been growing yearly more and more full of interest. As the hospital becomes more widely known we have a greater range of cases presenting themselves, and consequently have broader scope for usefulness ; and with the very efficient help now at our command, we are able to undertake surgical operations of great magnitude, which, while being causes of much anxiety, are also, when brought to a successful issue, reasons for profound thankfulness. If our Directors belonged largely to the medical fraternity, I should be tempted to become enthusiastic over some of the ' cases ' treated ; but this not being so, I will endeavour to keep my medical enthusiasm under proper control.

" *Private Practice amongst the Wealthy Classes.*—As many and various forms ot effort go to advance our common cause, I would like to draw attention to the good work accomplished this year by our chief medical assistant, Dr. Lin-luen-fai. He was one of the Government students sent to America to obtain a good English education. After his return he passed through the medical course in our school, and received his diploma, coming out first in his class. More than three years ago he was attached as a permanent assistant to aid in the hospital and school work, receiving from the Viceroy a salary of forty taels a month. In hospital and .dispensary practice you necessarily fail to reach large numbers of the wealthy and official classes. At the commencement of the Medical Mission in Tien-tsin I gave up a considerable share of my time to this depart-

ment—viz., visiting the wealthy in their own homes.
While resulting in much pecuniary gain to the hospital at
a time when such help was needed, yet the distances to
be travelled, and the cumbrous etiquette from which you
cannot in courtesy escape, absorb so much time, while the
spiritual results are so meagre, that I gradually withdrew
from it, and refused, except in very special cases, to visit
patients at their own abodes. But, though I thought my
time could be better employed, yet I consider such a line
of work as having a distinct value of its own. I have,
therefore, encouraged Dr. Lin to obtain as much private
practice as he can without interfering with his set duties.
During the year he has thus attended a large circle of the
educated and influential with much success ; notably one
gentleman, whose interest in our work on its philanthropic
side gives cause for true thankfulness. H. E. Yen-hsin-heu,
a Taotai in rank, and one of the wealthiest men in Tien-tsin,
now acting as chief director of the new Chinese Railway
Company, has been for many years friendly and sympa-
thetic. He was cured of chronic dysentery while under our
treatment, and was a subscriber to the original building
fund of the hospital, and later on to the extension fund.
Last summer, after a trying overland journey, he was
taken seriously ill with an acute affection of the heart
and other complications. He was so dangerously ill that
there seemed small hopes of his recovery ; however, Dr.
Lin visited him twice a day, paying the most assiduous
attention to his treatment, while I saw him at intervals,
and after many weeks of anxiety he was mercifully restored
to perfect health. A man of great influence in the city,
and justly popular, he was besieged during his severe
illness by many friends, who besought him to stop taking
foreign medicine, which might do well enough for foreign
constitutions, but could not be expected to suit the more
intricate anatomy of the Chinaman. However, the whole
gravity of the case, together with the nature of the lesion

and the object of the treatment, had been fully explained
to him—a questionably wise proceeding in ordinary
instances, but rendered necessary by the circumstances.
Mr. Yen, however, in spite of the opposition of his many
friends, preferred to trust himself in the hands of Dr. Lin,
and, happily, his trust was not misdirected. I should say,
by way of explanation, that in Tien-tsin, while Western
surgery is acknowledged as superior to Chinese, the same
does not hold good of the treatment of internal maladies.
One of the most earnest in entreating Mr. Yen to abandon
foreign physic was the present magistrate of the city, Mr.
Kung ; yet when the patient recovered, Dr. Lin received
a request to come and treat this magistrate's wife. Mr.
Yen's gratitude was very real. He not only presented two
commendatory tablets to be suspended outside the hospital,
—the ordinary method adopted by grateful patients,—but
he inserted, in the Chinese edition of the *Times* newspaper,
a paragraph expressing his indebtedness to Western medicine, and urging more of his countrymen to avail themselves
of it. He also memorialized the Viceroy to the same effect,
thanking him, as the patron of the hospital, for the benefits
he had received ; and within these last few days he has
appointed one of our old students to the post of medical
officer to the China Railway Company.

"*The Medical School.*—In December 1881 this small
school was started as an experiment. It was, and is, a
Government school, excepting that the foreign teachers are
medical missionaries. The idea of the scheme from the
Government point of view was to provide a few foreign
trained medical officers of the army and navy at a minimum
cost. The idea of the scheme from the missionary point
of view was to influence a band of educated young men
for Christ. It was hoped that it would be the beginning
of a much-needed medical college, with an efficient teaching
staff, and thoroughly furnished in all its branches. No
such institution exists in China, though an attempt is this

year being made in Hong Kong to found one under British auspices. Our hopes as to the growth of the school have not been realized, and we are compelled to acknowledge that, so far as the Chinese are concerned, we are ahead of the times. Chiefly due to the opposition shown by the officers in the army and navy to the innovation of foreign trained medical men, the interest in the growth of the school has largely ceased. Several of the late students have left the services dissatisfied with the treatment they were receiving, and the present ones are naturally greatly disheartened at the prospect awaiting them when they, too, a few months hence, will finish their course. The work of medical teaching is very onerous, and, although the authorities seem prepared to continue the school on its old footing, it appears to us wiser to add no more new students while the outlook for them is so poor.

" We cannot say that the experiment has failed, for from the Government standpoint they will have available, when the present class has got through, nineteen men who have undergone a three years' course in medicine upon the Western model, have studied Western text-books, and have been examined by Western practitioners. Nor from the missionary standpoint can the experiment be declared a failure. Sunday after Sunday, not to speak of the indirect influences during the week, the students have been under careful religious instruction, and we have had the joy of seeing several of them come out on the Lord's side. Let me mention an incident which greatly cheered my heart. The subject in our Bible class was the transfiguration on the mount. K. began the conversation by remarking, 'The three disciples saw the Lord in His glory, and we have now the like privilege. Last week,' said he, ' while I was reading and thinking over this lesson, I had a sort of vision. I saw Jesus as I had never seen Him before. I saw Him in His glory, and it made my heart so glad.' The young fellow gave this testimony before the class, evidently moved by the Spirit of God, for the Lord's presence was very manifest just then in our midst.

"Mr. King told me only yesterday an incident which may be worth recording. A friend spoke to him of a conversation he had had with Captain von Hanneken, a German officer in the Chinese service, who has had military command for nine years at Port Arthur, a fortified station at the mouth of the Gulf of Pechili. Dr. Chow, an old student, was in medical charge of the military hospital at the station, which was under the oversight of Captain von Hanneken. Speaking of Dr. Chow, who has since left the service and taken up a business appointment, the captain said that he had been badly treated by the Chinese officials at Port Arthur, though he himself had been greatly pleased with the young doctor. 'He did his work faithfully and well, and the only fault I had to find with him was that he read his Bible too much, and did not take sufficient exercise.'

"*Spiritual Results in the Hospital.*—In past years we have had cause to thank God for sending many material blessings; but, however stimulating to our faith these gifts may be when sent in answer to prayer, they only lead us the more hungrily to desire those spiritual blessings, the effect of which will·reach on into eternity. If last year was a good one in this latter respect—and we believe it was—this year has been a better. It may be safely said that there is a perceptible growth manifest in the spiritual life of our helpers. This is an omen of good things to come.

"In dealing with our patients we have aimed not only at the healing of their bodies, but at the salvation of their souls. Very many, thank God, have been attracted by the story of redemption, and not a few have thrown in their lot with us. Let me give a few instances :—

"Chang-te-Chun, aged thirty, a soldier. He was in hospital over two years ago undergoing a severe surgical operation. He made a good recovery, and during his con-

valescence became much interested in the gospel. Mani-
festing evidences of conversion, he was baptized in Tien-tsin
before his departure to his camp at Lu-tai, some two hundred
odd li from here.   He has paid us visits off and on as opportunity allowed, and has ever showed a warm love for the
Saviour and a desire to propagate the gospel.   On one
occasion he brought a subscription to be devoted to the
help of poor patients.   In the hospital gatehouse during
another visit he met a Bible colporteur, whom he invited
to visit Lu-tai.   The colporteur accepted the invitation, and
our soldier-friend gave him a hearty welcome.   He introduced him amongst his acquaintances, bore witness to the
truth, and in the public street urged the people to buy the
Scriptures and turn to the Saviour.   His aggressive Christianity brought upon him so much persecution in the camp,
where the men are generally the ruffians and ne'er-do-weels
who have found their own neighbourhoods too hot for
them, that after having received a severe beating from his
comrades he decided to leave the army.   In China, in time
of peace, no difficulty is thrown in the way of a soldier
leaving his regiment, as there are always more applicants
for enlistment than can be accepted, and his training
hitherto has not tended to make him a specially valuable
article in the market.   Though Chang-te-Chun left the
army, he did not leave Lu-tai ; but being a man of many
expedients, and having saved some money, he opened a
general shop in the town, and has since prospered.   He
continues as zealous as ever, and is a witness for Christ
in his district.   The Rev. Mr. Walker, of the American
Methodist Episcopal Mission, Tien-tsin, during a tour last
year, visited Lu-tai with the colporteur above referred to,
and remained a day or two preaching in the place.   He
told me he met two Christians there, both of whom had
been old patients, and he especially spoke in warm terms
of the earnestness of Mr. Chang, and of the help he had
received from him.   Mr. Chang brought two men, who had

been instructed by him, and who were hopeful inquirers, to see Mr. Walker.

"It is very difficult in China for a man to be a Christian and a soldier at the same time. Quite apart from the character of his comrades, he has to face the observance of idolatrous practices. Two or three times every year the 'cannon' are brought out for worship, offerings are presented, incense is burnt, and officers in turn prostrate themselves before the guns.

"What has been said of soldiers applies with still greater force to officers, whether civil or military. A blue-buttoned military mandarin, who was an in-patient, showed much interest in the gospel, and appeared to realize in some measure his need of a Saviour, but the consequences staring him in the face if he became a Christian were such that he shrank back. 'It would mean ruin to all my prospects,' said he, 'and I should have no rice to eat.'

"So with civil officials it practically means forsaking office to become a Christian. Two men of this class during the year were so far hopeful that they examined into the truth with apparently open minds, and in each case were considerably influenced. One was a Chow magistrate, and the other a grain official, both scholarly men, but the difficulty felt by each was, 'I cannot be a Christian and continue to hold my office.' Social ruin they thought would be the consequence, and they were not prepared to forsake all and follow Christ.

"Lin-tsung-lin, aged thirty-six, is a Nankin man, and the son of a sub-prefect. Though his rank is military, he has a good education and belongs to a good family. Such a combination is by no means common. Presumably for this reason he is not attached to the army, but is employed on the Viceroy's staff to fill special service appointments. Mr. Lin was an in-patient in the fourth month of the year, suffering from an affection of the elbow joint, which rendered his left arm useless. He made a complete recovery, with a useful arm. While with us he read the Scriptures and other books, and took a pleasure in conversing about Christianity. He had less pride than most men of his class, and was altogether a very lovable man. When he left, like so many more, he was undecided, and we could only leave him to God, not knowing what the result would be. However, he continued to attend Sunday services, and, having become an applicant for baptism, he was received in the tenth month. His friends proved his greatest hindrance, and for a time kept him back. Living in good style, and being an amiable man, he naturally had many friends. Some of them belonged to the order styled in China 'Chiu jou pêng yu,' which means literally 'wine and meat friends.' In this country such men are veritable leeches, and Mr. Lin found it no easy task to shake them oft. The early morning would find them in his guest room, and when he went abroad they would be at hand ready to escort him. Before his baptism he several times started to service or to visit us, but with his 'friends' dogging his steps he was ashamed to come. Then they began to insinuate that he was going over to the foreigner. To become a Christian is, with the wealthy Chinese, equivalent to becoming a *Kuri tzu nu,—i.e.*, a devil's slave—devil being the polite designation applied to the foreigner by the Chinese in their own homes. It was his good old mother —all honour to the old lady—who at last came to the rescue, and gave the so-called friends a thorough rating, declaring that her son was doing no disgraceful act in joining the foreign religion. From this time he took a more decided stand. He threw away his ancestral tablet, and cleared all trace of idolatry from his house. His old mother, over sixty years of age, who reads well, is much interested in the gospel, having been instructed by her son, and having studied the New Testament for herself. A manservant in his employ is also under instruction.

"Kêng-lien-Chen, aged thirty, pedlar. He was converted

when in the hospital two years ago. He carried on his calling for some time in Tien-tsin, and was received into the Church. Needing a hospital coolie, and wishing to have a Christian man, about seven months since we engaged the pedlar. He gave great satisfaction, as he devoted nearly all his spare time to teaching the patients what he himself knew; and as he had a good knowledge of characters, and was well acquainted with his New Testament, he was a great help. About a month ago he asked permission to leave, as he felt it on his conscience to return to his home at Laoling, some three hundred li from Tien-tsin, and preach the gospel to his relations and neighbours. ' Go, by all means,' said I, for I much wish that more of the Christians had it in their hearts to go and tell others what God has done for their souls. I trust he may be sustained and blest in his mission.

"We have had the privilege of seeing what comfort Christianity brings during the last moments of life, in two cases dying in hospital within the year. One had served the Lord for some years in the capacity of native preacher in the American Methodist Episcopal Mission. He became an in-patient for acute inflammation of the bowels, which led to the formation of an abscess, and the cutting short of his promising career at the age of thirty-nine. Mr. Wang-chih-ho always had a bright and happy smile to greet one upon entering his ward, and you felt, while conversing with him, that Christianity did indeed mean to him faith in a living Christ. The day before he died, though there were no special symptoms to denote that the end was coming, he himself realized that death was close at hand; yet, with this presentiment, God graciously sent calmness and peace of heart. On this day, after one of the dispensers had been speaking as usual to the patients in his ward, Mr. Wang addressed them, and spoke of his expectation of death and of the certain hope he had of life eternal in Christ Jesus. His words were accompanied with spiritual power, and, while speaker and listener wept together, those who were able knelt upon the floor while the dying believer prayed for God's blessing upon them.

"Another case was that of Wang-san, aged twenty-eight, who entered the hospital in 1886, suffering from chronic disease of the knee-joint, which totally disabled him. As a last resource, excision of the knee-joint was performed under antiseptic precautions, and he was able to get about again. But his constitution had been shattered by his long illness, and he died in the hospital eight months after the operation was performed. Upon his first coming under our care he was very callous and indifferent to everything but his sickness; this condition lasted for about a month, during which time it seemed well-nigh hopeless to move his heart, but he awoke at last to a sense of his sinfulness and need of a Saviour. When he got about again, after the operation, he was baptized, and proved himself a simple-minded, warm-hearted Christian. Not knowing a character when he first came in, he could, at the time of his death, read his New Testament fairly well, which speaks highly for his interest and perseverance. At ten o'clock at night, four hours before his death, I sat on the side of his kang; he was evidently sinking, yet his mind was quite clear, and we talked together of the life beyond the grave. He was quite restful and happy—his was a simple faith, but oh, you could not doubt its potency as you saw his face lit up with the radiance of hope. After prayer together I wished him good-bye, not expecting he would live until morning. His last words to me were, 'Doctor, I shall be waiting for you in heaven; I am going on before.' This man, a year previously, had been dark and dead in heathenism, now he was a new creature in Christ Jesus. As I went to my room I thought to myself, 'Oh, this is indeed worth coming to China for!'"

The Doctor's last letter to his father is dated March 20th, less than a fortnight before his death

"I hope you are all keeping well," he writes. "Alec tells me you are getting on nicely in the trying January weather.

"Now business life has come back to Tien-tsin with the opening of the river and the arrival of the steamers. The opening up of the inland rivers also increases my work, as a large number of country people, who were not able to travel in the winter by road, now come long distances very cheaply by boat.

"These cases are chiefly surgical ones of long standing coming in for operation. We have a large number of in-patients just now, and they are, quite a lot of them, interested in the gospel and studying their Bibles and catechisms. You would be interested in the sight going on in the wards nearly every afternoon—little groups of patients gathered round one or two beds, and one of the hospital helpers busy teaching them.

"Would that God would pour down a very great blessing on the hospital this year. There is certainly no such field for evangelistic work as the wards of an hospital in a land like China, where it is well-nigh impossible to come in touch with the people.

"It is very wonderful to see how step by step God has opened up this work, and is now using it to spread into all the districts around the precious word of salvation.

"Dr. Roberts has gone to join Gilmour in Mongolia, and the Macfarlanes are in the country, with Mr. Rees, arranging their new home. I am therefore all alone."

During the days that followed the writing of these letters Dr. Mackenzie's time was even more fully occupied than usual, for of him it might be truly said that he died in harness. Sickness was very prevalent throughout the settlement of Tien-tsin, and the only medical man then residing in the place had been summoned to Taku, at the mouth of the river, to attend some patients who were seriously ill with small pox. As was his custom, Dr. Irwin had left his practice in Dr. Mackenzie's hands, so that he had a time of exceptionally hard work. It is possible that from this cause he may have been predisposed to sickness, but was apparently in perfect health when, on Saturday afternoon, he attended as usual the weekly meeting of the Chinese and foreign workers connected with the Mission, for prayer and consultation.

He afterwards took a walk over the plain with Mr. King. The weather had been unseasonably warm during the week, and consequently heavy winter clothing had been pretty generally laid aside. One of the cold bleak winds for which our northern springs are distinguished suddenly came up, and Dr. Mackenzie, having neglected to take with him his overcoat, took a severe chill. On the next day, though evidently suffering from cold, he attended as usual both Chinese and English services. He had arranged to dine with one of the Mission families, and had the pleasure of meeting with his friends Mr. and Mrs. Pigott, of the China Inland Mission, who had just returned to China after furlough, and were passing through Tien-tsin to their station in the interior.

How little we thought it was the last Sabbath he would spend on earth. He talked cheerfully and brightly of the medical work, when questioned by Mr. Pigott. In reply to enquiries made, with some surprise, as to his intention of closing the medical school when the students then in the classes had graduated, he replied, that after much thought and prayer about the matter, he felt convinced it was the right thing to do, since the need for such trained medical men was not yet felt in China, except spasmodically, in times of special emergency, when rumours of war were abroad.

"Will you, then, refuse students if they are sent to you by the Viceroy?" enquired his friend.

"His Excellency is not likely to send me any, unless I make the request," he replied.

Being further pressed as to how he would make his decision known to the Viceroy, he explained, "I have never troubled myself about the future; that is in God's hands; He will make all clear when the time comes."

Some conversation was also carried on about the Anti-Vivisection Society in England, with some ardent members of which his friends had met while at home.

Dr. Mackenzie considered that it was possible to push this matter too far, and related how a lady at home had refused to shake hands with him, because he could not conscientiously say that he believed vivisection of every kind and under any circumstances was to be condemned.

After conducting his afternoon Bible class, he attended the English service, and then took supper with his old friends Mr. and Mrs. Innocent, of the Methodist New Connexion Mission. They thought him feverish and far from well, but no serious illness was anticipated.

The fever increased, but after a restless night the Doctor rose, and went to the dispensary as usual. His strength was, however, not equal to his desire to work, and he was compelled to leave the place where he had laboured so nobly and successfully, for the last time, and go back to his bedchamber. At five o'clock on Monday afternoon, the hour of our weekly prayer-meeting, two of the members of the Mission were absent. Just at the close Mr. Bryson came in and informed us of the Doctor's serious illness. On his way from the city he had been met by one of the dispensers, who had told him that Dr. Mackenzie was very ill, and the fever rising. Upon going up to his room Dr. Mackenzie remarked to his colleague, " I am afraid this is going to be something rather serious, I have never felt anything like it before."

He was asked if he would like to have Dr. Irwin called in, and upon giving his assent, that gentleman was at once summoned.

Both doctors were agreed in fearing the disease threatened might be small pox, as Dr. Mackenzie had been attending patients suffering from that epidemic.

When we heard this sad news, before the prayer-
meeting broke up we all joined in earnest supplication, that if it were the Lord's will the disease might
be rebuked, and our dear friend's valuable life
spared.

The next two days there seemed little change in
the patient's condition. Mr. and Mrs. King kindly
acted as nurses, with the help of some of the Doctor's
students, and to guard against risk of contagion every
one else was, by the Doctor's orders, excluded from the
room.

From that time Dr. Mackenzie seemed to entertain
no thoughts of recovery. Dr. Irwin was anxious
about this impression, and constantly reminded his
patient that they had both attended more serious
cases where recovery had supervened.

Frequent interviews and excitement were forbidden
by the doctor in attendance, but Dr. Mackenzie's two
senior colleagues kept watch for several nights in the
room below his bedchamber.

On Good Friday morning Mr. Lees was allowed
to see his sick friend, and he at once asked him to
pray with him. Allusion being made in the prayer
to the sacred memories of the day, the Doctor enquired,
" Is this Good Friday then ? " and seemed from the
expression of his face to derive pleasure from the
fact, as if in some way it brought him nearer to his
Lord. Our " beloved physician " had heard the call
which summoned him to rest from his labours, and
when another colleague entered the room he ex-

claimed, " I think the Lord is calling me to Himself. What a joy it will be to go to Him ! What a mercy to be prepared to go."

Another pathetic incident of that morning was Dr. Mackenzie's parting with one of the ablest of his staff, a man of high character and attainments, who has long been a Christian man, but whose lukewarmness has lately given us cause for anxiety. Fixing his eyes upon him, he said with great solemnity :—

" Ah, sir, when it comes to this there is no peace, no rest, for a man but in Jesus ! Don't let the world get hold of you. Don't let anxiety to please your worldly friends, and the cares and honours of the world, drive you away from Jesus. I am afraid for you." And then, as, speechless with grief, the man turned to go, he held out his hand, and on his Chinese friend taking it in sign of farewell, he added, " Whether we shall meet again or not is for you to decide."

It was on the afternoon of this day that Dr. Irwin first expressed fears as to the issue, and about one o'clock on Saturday morning Dr. Mackenzie sent for Mr. Lees to speak to him about his will and receive parting messages for friends. He was then in great pain, but it was characteristic of him that his sole anxiety was that everything should be clearly explained, so as to save trouble when he was gone.

The night was one of great distress, owing to increased difficulty of breathing, and in the morning, when Mr. Lees saw him again, he said,—

" Oh, I have had such a dreadful night. I cannot

bear this much longer. Do pray the Lord to call me away soon."

A little later he said, " I felt a presentiment on Monday when I became ill. One does not usually lay any stress on presentiments, but I had the feeling that this would be my last illness."

" I hope not," replied his colleague. " I trust that God will spare you to us for many years yet. We want you, and the Lord's work wants you."

" Oh, it is all right," replied the Doctor. " I am quite ready to go."

Some relief was experienced towards the afternoon of Saturday ; the breathing seemed easier, and though the inflammation had not begun to subside, it was understood that the right lung was still not affected. It was arranged that Mrs. Lees should watch over the patient during the night, in company with two of the Doctor's attached medical students.

We all retired to rest with the strain of intense anxiety somewhat relieved, and were daring to hope that the crisis had passed, and that the morning might see some marked improvement in our dear friend's condition.

Towards midnight Dr. Irwin left him, feeling more encouraged about the case.

Dr. Mackenzie seemed easier and inclined for conversation, but Mrs. Lees rather discouraged this, fearing the least excitement might produce unfavourable symptoms. He enquired what Dr. Irwin thought of his condition, and Mrs. Lees replied that he con-

sidered there was a slight change for the better, and
that we hoped God was going to spare him to us
to do some more work for the Master.

"You would like that, would you not?" she
enquired.

"Yes," he said; "I am quite ready, whichever way
it is. I only want the Lord's will to be done. It
would be nice to stay and do a little more work, if
that is His will."

Then, at a suggestion from Mrs. Lees that he
had better try and get a little sleep, he turned over
on his side, remarking, "Oh, this is so restful; I feel
as if I could sleep so well for such a long time."

For some time he seemed to be peacefully sleeping,
till suddenly, about twenty minutes to four, the heavy
breathing suddenly stopped. One of the students,
who had been watching outside the door, instantly
noticed the change, and, coming in, at once felt his
pulse, and discovered that thus silently and peacefully
he had gone to be for ever with the Lord.

There seemed to be something specially beautiful
in the time of his release. "Very early in the morning,
while it was yet dark," on Easter Day, "God's finger
touched him, and he slept;" and with the news of the
great sorrow which had fallen upon us as a Mission,
came thoughts of all that the glorious Resurrection
morning signifies to sorrowing hearts down all the
ages.

But the loss was felt to be indeed a heavy one
both by Chinese and foreigners. Seldom, perhaps,

has any one been called away from one of our
Eastern communities whose death has been so
universally mourned, as his who might well be
called "the beloved physician."

Throughout the native city, from the home of
the Viceroy to the humble abode of many a poor
coolie, to whom the skilful hand, now cold in death,
had brought relief and healing, the news that one so
honoured and beloved had passed away was received
with dismay and heartfelt sorrow. " He was indeed
a good man and a skilful ; " " There will never be such
another physician ! " " How can the sick be healed
now ? "—such were a few of the expressions that
might be heard falling from Chinese lips as the sad
news that " Ma Tai-fu " was dead spread through the
city. And not among the Chinese alone, but in
many a foreign home, where in times of sickness
life and health had been restored by his skill, and
hope rekindled by the confidence his presence inspired in every patient's heart, there also his loss
was mourned as no common sorrow.

The funeral took place on the afternoon of the
day following his death, only a week from the
commencement of his illness.

It was a lovely afternoon, the air balmy and
warm, and fragrant with the breath of peach
blossoms,—a great contrast to the bleak dust storms
and leaden skies of the day on which the beloved
departed lay dying.

Very striking was the wonderful burst of spontancous feeling which affected our cosmopolitan community, and brought men of every nationality in unprecedented numbers to show their respect by attendance at the funeral. Large crowds of Chinese, whose special friend he was, thronged the road to the cemetery, in many cases evidently mourning the loss of one to whom they had been sincerely attached.

"I never thought Chinamen could be so affected," remarked one, who saw the marks of deep and heart-felt sorrow on many a Chinese face, as they stood by Dr. Mackenzie's open grave.

Borne by Chinese dispensers and Christians, the coffin was carried from the Doctor's home to the little English church not far distant. It was almost covered by beautiful wreaths and garlands of choice flowers from the greenhouses of English, German, and Russian friends, mingled with the humbler floral offerings of many others who had known and loved him. Among these last gifts of love glittered the Star and Ribbon of the Double Dragon, conferred upon Dr. Mackenzie by the Emperor a few years previously.

The coffin was borne up the aisle of the little church past crowds of mourners of all nationalities, conspicuous among them being two high officers, deputed by Lady Li and the Viceroy to represent them.

Suddenly the beautiful strains of the "Christian's Good-night" were raised; a sweet expression of the

24

comfort which comes to the mourners of those who have fallen asleep in Jesus.

> " Sleep on, belovéd, sleep and take thy rest,
>   Lay down thy head upon thy Saviour's breast;
>   We love thee well, but Jesus loves thee best.
>   Good-night.
>
> " Until the shadows from this earth are cast,
>   Until He gathers in His sheaves at last,
>   Until the twilight gloom is overpast,
>   Good-night.
>
> " Until the Easter glory lights the skies,
>   Until the dead in Jesus shall arise,
>   And He shall come, but not in lowly guise,
>   Good-night.
>
> " Only 'Good-night,' belovéd, not ' Farewell; '
>   A little while, and all His saints shall dwell
>   In hallowed union indivisible.
>   Good-night.
>
> " Until we meet again before the Throne,
>   Clothed in the spotless robe He gives His own,
>   Until we know even as we are known,
>   Good-night."

The short service in the church was conducted by the Rev. J. Innocent, of the English Methodist New Connexion Mission.

The coffin was borne from thence to the end of the road leading to the cemetery by twelve friends, including gentlemen of the foreign community and the representatives of seven missions, some of whom, it happened, at that time were passing through Tientsin on their way to interior stations.

From the end of the cemetery road to the grave
the bearers were twelve of Dr. Mackenzie's medical
students, who, at their own special request, were
allowed the privilege of rendering this last service to
their departed teacher.

An impressive service was conducted at the grave-
side by the Rev. J. Lees, the senior representative
of the London Mission in Tien-tsin, a portion of it
being in Chinese for the benefit of the large concourse
of native Christians who attended. Then the well-
known strains of the hymn "Rock of Ages" were
raised, sounding familiar even in its Chinese garb,
and bringing back to many a heart touching memories
of sacred services in the homeland so far away, the
land to which the day before the sad and startling
tidings of their heavy loss had been flashed to the
aged father, the widow, and little child. A shadow
seemed to have fallen over the lives of not a few,
as we turned away from Dr. Mackenzie's early
grave.

Could it be true that he, little more than a week
ago so full of life and vigour, was now numbered
with the dead, having been called away from the
work for which he seemed so peculiarly fitted? How
was it that he had been called to rest from his
labours, when the Master's injunction that we should
pray for more labourers to be sent into His harvest-
field seemed more incumbent upon us than ever
before?

That he had in truth been called to higher service

was the thought of many a heart, while the question
of Dean Alford,

> " Who knoweth if to live be but to die,
>   And death be life ? "

echoed through our thoughts.

There, in the quiet churchyard in the land of his
adoption, among the people whom he loved and
lived for, the tired body lies sleeping ; but we cannot
but believe that the active soul has found a higher
sphere of service in that land where it is said, " His
servants shall serve Him."

" The future world," writes General Gordon, " has
been somehow painted to our minds as a place of
continuous praise, and though we may not say it,
we cannot help feeling that if thus it would prove
monotonous. It cannot be thus. It must be a life
of activity ; death is cessation of movement, life is all
movement."

> " The tasks, the joys of earth, the same in heaven will be,
>   Only the little brook has widened to a sea,"

sings Archbishop Trench, and our hearts are inclined
to feel as if he may be more nearly right than we
know.

At any rate, we feel that the influence of such a life
as Dr. Mackenzie's does not end when the grave
covers him from our sight.

Such men, it has well been said, " create an epidemic
of nobleness ; " and though it is true that we can only
gaze with profit upon God's saints in so far as they

dimly reflect the image of their Saviour, we know
well that "men do become wiser and greater by
gazing at such examples, more ready to do and dare,
more willing to lift their eyes out of the mire of
selfishness and the dust of anxiety and toil, more
brave to try whether they too cannot scale the
toppling crags of duty and hold converse with these
their loftier brethren upon

> ' the shining tablelands
> To which our God Himself is moon and sun.' " *

And it was not merely an enthusiasm for humanity
that touched Mackenzie's heart and made him willing
to give up his life for the benefit of the millions of
China. Men have done noble deeds under the
stimulus of philanthropy, but a higher motive than
this was the mainspring of his life, and that was
a consuming love for his Divine Master. Like St.
Paul, he was willing to become a fool for Christ's
sake, and not a few men of the world so regarded
him. For they saw that with many opportunities for
enriching himself he accumulated no fortune; that
although he might have yielded to the temptations to
vanity which recognised ability and success place in a
man's way, he yet grew more humble with the passing
years, while he curbed and mastered a naturally hasty
temper till men wondered at his calmness.

How striking was the testimony of a Chinaman
who had known him intimately for years. While the

---

* Farrar.

Doctor lay dying this man remarked, " I believe in
Dr. Mackenzie. He is a true man and a real follower
of Christ. We talk of getting rid of our faults, and I
suppose we all do try more or less earnestly to do so,
but I have known very few men who have really
much changed. Dr. Mackenzie has. Good as he was
when I first knew him, he has become better ; he
has become humble and patient, and has gained
control over his temper. Yes, he has grown more like
Jesus."

The Doctor had made it a matter of special prayer
that the year of which he only lived three short
months should be a time of very special blessing
to the hospital. It seemed a strange answer to this
petition, that in so short a time he who had been the
very mainspring of the work should have been removed
from it. But God's ways are not as our ways, and
His thoughts are higher than our thoughts. " He
buries His workmen, but he carries on His work."

A few short months after Dr. Mackenzie's death
saw the hospital entirely stripped of all the temporal
advantages and pecuniary help it had so long enjoyed,
with the patronage of the Viceroy and high officials
entirely withdrawn from it.

The reserve fund, which with so much diligence
and economy Dr. Mackenzie had accumulated through
many years, and which he believed would be the
means, not only of supporting the Tien-tsin medical
work in the future, but also of supplying the funds
for opening dispensaries and hospitals in needy

districts throughout Northern China, was wrested from the Mission. The London Missionary Society was merely allowed the option of purchasing the buildings in which Dr. Mackenzie had for so many years carried on his noble and beneficent work. Meanwhile the Chinese authorities opened a Government Naval Hospital in close proximity to what had been known as the Viceroy's Hospital, but will henceforth bear the name of the London Mission.

Yet all this failed materially to injure the work which had been founded and baptized in believing prayer. More than two years have passed since Dr. Mackenzie's death, and during that time the work has been carried on as successfully as before. God Himself sent us a physician likeminded with Dr. Mackenzie. The sick attend at the dispensary in larger numbers even than before. The hospital wards have been well filled, while the spiritual blessings which in years past have distinguished the hospital as a nursery of the Church have still been vouchsafed to us by the Lord of the harvest.

As to the pecuniary needs of the work, the Lord who gave and afterwards saw fit to take away the patronage of the rich and great Chinese officials, has been pleased to supply what has been needed from time to time, by putting it into the hearts of His people, both here and in the homeland, to contribute to the necessities of the work upon which His smile still rests.

As to the further results of Dr. Mackenzie's

labours in quarters in which, while still with us, he felt somewhat discouraged, the following extract from the present year's report of Dr. Roberts, who succeeded Dr. Mackenzie in the Tien-tsin medical work, shows that even here his earnest labours are bringing forth fruit as the years pass by.

"You will be glad to know," he writes, "that the former labours of our lamented brother, Dr. Mackenzie, in connection with the Government medical school under his charge, have been far from fruitless. Up to the time of his death it seemed to him almost like labour in vain, seeing that the graduates were not succeeding in obtaining appointments.

"It is very different now. In close proximity to our own hospital is an imposing building, the Viceroy's hospital, managed for the most part by three of Dr. Mackenzie's former students, and with the prospect, if well conducted, of doing much good in the healing of the sick. In Port Arthur there is a naval and military hospital and dispensary, which is much appreciated by the soldiers, and it is also worked by former students. Others again have been appointed to Wei Hai Wei, a naval station. Dr. Chang has been accepted many months ago for the post of house surgeon to the Alice Memorial Hospital, Hong-Kong; while last, but not least, Dr. Mai has been for some time successfully treating the father of the Emperor in Peking."

APPENDIX.

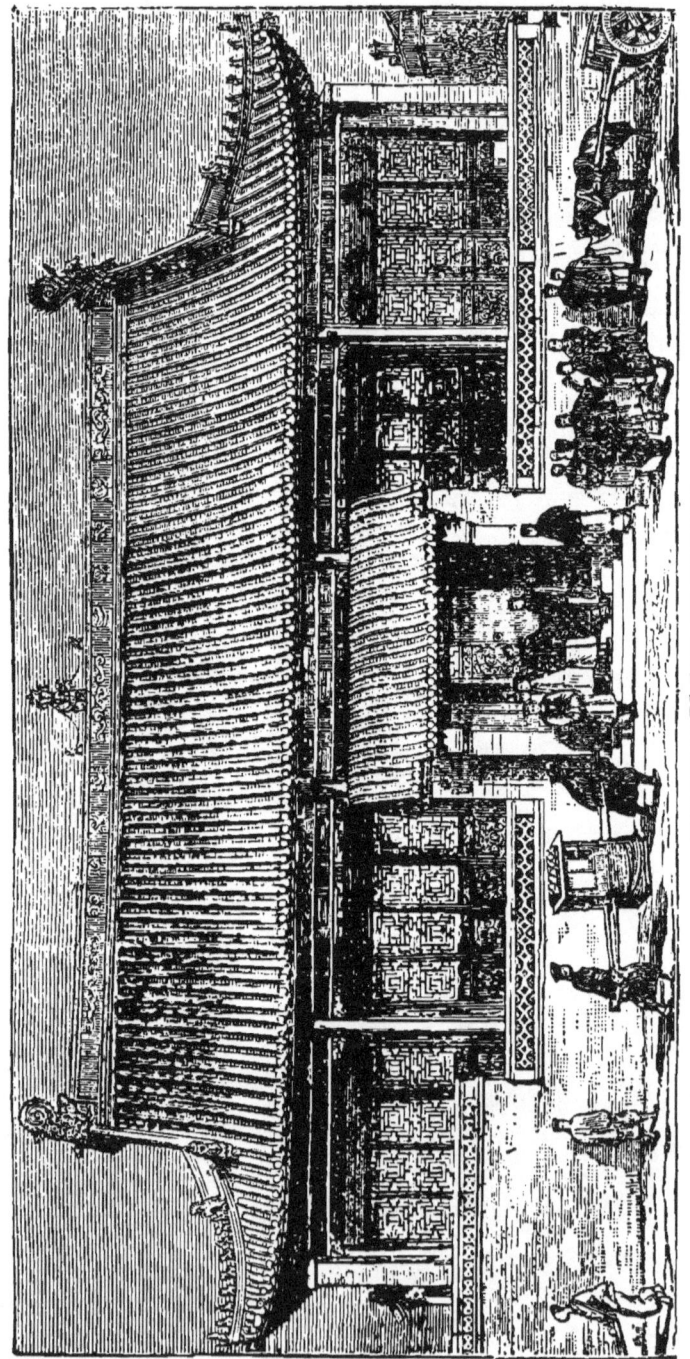

THE NEW HOSPITAL AT TIEN-TSIN.

I.

NORTH CHINA.—NEW HOSPITAL AT TIEN-TSIN.

BY J. KENNETH MACKENZIE, M.R.C.S.

THE new hospital on the London Mission Compound, commenced in the autumn of 1879, is now completed, and was publicly opened on Thursday, December 2nd, by His Excellency Li Hung Chang, Viceroy of the Metropolitan Province, Imperial Grand Secretary, etc. The occasion was one of special interest, in that it elicited the hearty co-operation of both Chinese and foreigners. The hospital is built on the east side of the Taku Road, the main thoroughfare between the native city and the foreign concession and shipping. It is erected in the best style of Chinese architecture, and has an extremely picturesque and attractive appearance. The front building, standing in its own courtyard, is raised six or seven feet above the level of the road, and is ascended by broad stone steps, which lead from the covered gateway to a verandah with its massive wooden pillars running along its whole length. A hall divides the building into two portions. On the right side and in front is a spacious dispensary, which, thanks to the liberality of the Viceroy, is wanting in nothing, rivalling any English dispensary in the abundance and variety of the drugs, appliances, etc.; behind this is a roomy drug store. On the left of the hall is a large waiting-room, with benches for the convenience of the patients, and used on Sundays and other days as a preaching hall. Behind and to one side is the usual Chinese reception-room ever to be found in a native building. Two other ante-rooms adjacent complete this block. The rooms are very lofty, without ceilings, leaving exposed the huge painted beams, many times larger than foreigners deem necessary, but the pride of the Chinese builder. Running off in two parallel wings at the back, each entirely detached and separated by courtyards, are the surgery and wards, the latter able to accommodate thirty-six in-patients. The wards to the right wing, four in number, are small, intended each to receive only three patients. Here we can isolate dangerous cases, and also receive persons, such as officials and others, who require greater privacy. In the left wing is the large ward, with accommodation for twenty-four patients, and beyond this a kitchen and other offices. The wards are all furnished with kangs, instead of beds, as is the custom in North China. These kangs are built with bricks, with flues running underneath, so that in winter they can be heated ; the bedding is spread upon a mat over the warm bricks. Plenty of room has been left for further extensions if found necessary.

The opening ceremony was a very interesting one. The various rooms were gaily decorated with flowers, shrubs, flags, etc. Men from the English and Chinese gunboats helped Mr. Lees and Mr. King in the work of transforming the rooms from their normal bareness into a right gala appearance. While the place of honour was reserved for the Chinese dragon, the other national flags were attached together, and drawn from beam to beam, making ceilings of variegated colours for the principal rooms ; the walls were also draped with bunting. The waiting-room, where the ceremony was to take place, was arranged as a Chinese grand reception-hall ; everything in it was native, borrowed from the yamens. The floor was covered with camels'-hair carpets, brought from the temple for the occasion. The drug store, empty of drugs, and in its gala dress, was laid out with tables spread with refreshments, arranged by the ladies of the Mission. Every delicacy in the way of cakes, fruit, etc., was provided for the guests. The courtyard was matted in, and the whole place hung with handsome Chinese lanterns.

By the appointed time all the Chinese and foreign guests had arrived, amongst them the three Taotais, the Prefect of the city, and numerous civil and military mandarins. Of the foreigners, the consular body was represented by the English, German, Russian, and American Consuls, officers from the ships of war, all the members of the missionary body, and many others.

Upon the arrival of His Excellency an illuminated address in Chinese was read and presented. The Viceroy, upon receiving it, uttered many kindly words, showing his appreciation of, and sympathy with, the work already done —" while disclaiming any praise or merit as due to himself in the matter, he took the opportunity of publicly expressing his thanks to me and warm approbation of the zeal with which foreign medical skill has been so freely bestowed upon the people of Tien-tsin."

Speeches were then made by Henry B. Bristow, Esq., H.B.M. Consul, and C. Waeber, Esq., Consul for Russia. Mr. Bristow spoke as follows : "It gives all foreigners the greatest pleasure to see His Excellency, the Grand Secretary, acting as patron of an institution like the one just opened. His Excellency has already gained great fame as a military commander, and it is to be hoped that in the future he would be also renowned for his encouragement of Western medical science. The reminiscences of military triumphs must always be embittered by the thoughts of friends killed, provinces devastated, crops destroyed, and all the evils which make war a curse to both victors and vanquished ; but the recollections associated with the establishment of benevolent institutions like the present brought to the mind only thoughts of pain assuaged and misery alleviated, and therefore he felt sure that His Excellency, when looking back

in years to come on his last achievements, would dwell with
more unmixed pleasure on the establishment of institutions
like the present than even on his military successes in the
service of his country."

Mr. C. Waeber, Russian Consul, also spoke, and said
that "we have a proverb, ' in corpore sano mens sana,'
which may be rendered in Chinese by ' T'i wang tsê shên
ch'ing'—When the body is vigorous, then the mind is
bright. In this new hospital we have a proof of His
Excellency's great care for the welfare of his people, and
it permits me to hope that His Excellency will take further
steps for the development of this country by introducing
Western art and science." Mr. Taotai Mah, Chief Secretary,
replied for the Viceroy in French, stating again what His
Excellency had already said in Chinese, and thanking all
present for their interest in the good work.

After the speaking had concluded, the native assistants
were introduced to the Viceroy. The Viceroy, having
formally opened the building, commenced a careful inspection; he examined many varieties of drugs, inquiring
into their properties, etc.; wanting to know if we had any
remedies in common with the Chinese; whether most of
our medicinal agents came from the organic or inorganic
kingdoms; as to the cost of foreign drugs, and other
queries too numerous to mention. But in the surgery the
greatest amount of interest was excited; the walls were
hung with anatomical and physiological charts, kindly lent
by Mrs. Williamson, of Chefoo; on the operating-table and
shelves were spread the valuable collection of surgical instruments belonging to the hospital, with models of the
human body and heart, lent by the Tien-tsin civil doctors.
Everything in this department was new, even to those
high officials, such as the Viceroy and Superintendent of
Arsenals, to whom the latest inventions in electricity and
mechanics are immediately sent. [It will probably surprise
many to know that, although there is no railroad in China,

His Excellency is better acquainted with the working of the steam-engine than most well-informed foreigners, having studied it intelligently from models.] Questions without number as to the uses, action, etc., of various instruments were put, and required all one's readiness of mind to give answers that would be easily comprehended. The size of the human brain in relation to the body, as shown in the wax model, drew special attention. The wards were afterwards examined, and the working of the hospital carefully inquired into.

The Viceroy and the other guests then sat down to the refreshments already provided. It was evident, as each took his departure at the close, that a very pleasant afternoon had been spent.

The Scheme Purely Chinese.—Medical mission hospitals in China have hitherto been mainly, if not altogether, supported by foreigners, the few occasional subscriptions obtained from the Chinese forming so small a proportion of the funds used in the carrying on of these various institutions as to be practically of but little account. We have, therefore, had an unique experience in Tien-tsin, in that the hospital has been built entirely with Chinese subscriptions, and the working expenses obtained from the same source. We would humbly acknowledge the goodness of God in the entire matter. He, of a truth, has heard and answered prayer, and where the door seemed well-nigh closed He has opened wide its portals. On the Sunday following the opening, December 5th, a praise meeting was held in the large waiting-room of the hospital, attended by members of all the churches in Tien-tsin. Rev. J. Lees presided, and, after an opening address, called upon Rev. J. Innocent, New Connexion Methodist; Rev. W. L. Pilcher, American Episcopal Methodist Mission; Rev. H. Porter, M.D., American Board, and myself, who all spoke in words of praise and thanksgiving for what God had manifestly wrought. Much prayer was offered up that, as God had already given so many temporal blessings, and drawn the people so near us, He would, in the days that are to come, pour down richly of those spiritual blessings for which our hearts are longing.

The Medical Mission accounts stand roughly as follow :—

Received from Viceroy for salaries of native helpers, purchase of surgical instruments, drugs, medical stores, and all expenses at temple dispensary and new hospital for fifteen months, ending November 30th, 1880 ... ... Tls. 4,000 = £1,200.

The above amount has been placed in the hands of W. W. Pethick, Esq., Secretary to His Excellency, and myself, who are jointly responsible for its use. The Viceroy has not been asked to contribute to the Building Fund.

BUILDING FUND.

Subscriptions to Building Fund from Chinese
to December 27th, 1880 ... ... Tls. 3,820 = £1,146
Sale of Medicines and Appliances to Chinese 500 =

Tls. 4,320 = £1,296

Amount paid to Builder ... ... 4,000 = 1,200
Balance in hand ... ... 320 = 96

From Viceroy and general subscribers, the total amount received, entirely from native sources, tls. 8,320 = £2,496 during the sixteen months.

The new hospital has already received over 200 in-patients, all of whom find their own food and clothing. Out-patients are still seen by me at the Memorial Temple four days a week. The register there shows the names of over 5,000 patients, with more than 20,000 visits.

II.

A MEDICAL REVIEW OF DR. MACKENZIE'S WORK.

It has been thought that a few lines on the medical aspect of the late Dr. Mackenzie's work might prove interesting to some of his medical friends, and also helpful to any who may be preparing for medical mission work in China. It is with this hope that we now record the leading facts, knowing well, however, that only an approximate idea can be thus gathered of the amount of suffering relieved and of the high professional value of the work of our lamented colleague.

Before referring to the various reports which Dr. Mackenzie published, and before the reader forms an opinion as to their value, it is necessary to bear in mind the numerous barriers to success which Dr. Mackenzie, in common with almost every medical missionary in China, had to contend with. These difficulties show us clearly the need of thorough preparation before coming to the Mission field.

First we note the extremely chronic nature of many of the cases treated. The reason is not far to seek. Many diseases which are amenable to treatment based on a knowledge of the anatomy, physiology, and pathology of the body, must necessarily, in a large measure, remain beyond the scope of the native physician, as he is practically ignorant of these sciences.

In addition to this, we must add the great distrust and prejudice still existing in the native mind, though to a less extent than in former years, in · consequence of which a Chinaman will often choose to endure months or even years of suffering rather than seek help from the foreign doctor.

A very real hindrance often presents itself in the insanitary hospital surroundings, and we are often powerless to improve matters. The hospital in Tien-tsin is an example of this, being surrounded by numerous graves and inundated plains,—a fruitful source of ague from time to time. In view

25

of these facts, we are not surprised at the need Mackenzie felt of thorough antiseptic precautions in order to success in operative surgery.

By looking over the Doctor's Annual Reports we may learn much as to the nature of his work, the varieties of diseases treated, as well as their relative frequency.

STATISTICS OF WORK IN HANKOW.

Year.	No. of Out-door Patients.	No. of In-door Patients.	No. of Operations.*
1876	3,128	93	55
1877	5,214	406	75
1878	11,859	1,137	123
Total	20,201	1,636	253

* Exclusive of opening abscesses and sinuses.

STATISTICS OF THE RELATIVE FREQUENCY OF THE COMMONER DISEASES MET WITH AMONG THE OUT-DOOR PATIENTS.

Year.	Chronic Rheumatism.	Scabies.	Conjunctivitis.	Eczema.	Malarial Fever.	Syphilis.	Granl. Conjunctivitis.
1876	277	228	336	140	51	111	122
1877	564	595	422	166	170	108	46
Total	841	823	758	306	221	219	168

The 253 operations performed in Hankow may be taken as representative of the nature of the surgical work which falls to a medical missionary in his early years of service. We notice that operations on the eye for cataract, pterygium, entropion, and iridectomy, are more numerous than any others; next come the excision of tumours, one of which weighed twenty-five pounds, and was successfully removed, the patient making a good recovery. Hare-lip cases were fairly numerous, but vesicle calculus was only met with four times; the lateral perineal operation was the one adopted for removal. We mention this latter fact as it presents a striking contrast to the great frequency of this disease in South China, particularly Canton and its neighbourhood.

Reference has been made, in a previous part of the memoir, to several medical and surgical cases of general interest, and to the Doctor's mode of solving the boarding problem among in-door patients. It alone remains to refer to his opium refuge work, and the views he held concerning the opium smoking habit.

We are all familiar with the difference of opinion held by medical men on this subject. Medical missionaries, some of whom speak from the personal observation of thousands of cases gathered from all grades of society, are unanimous in condemning the practice from a medical and moral stand-point, though at the same time they allow that in the case of the robust and well-to-do the physical harm may be slight compared with the degrading or at least hurtful moral effects on the victim of the pipe.

On the other hand it is surprising to find some medical men stating that the habit is practically harmless. That they think so conscientiously we doubt not, though we are at a loss to understand how they arrive at their conclusions—conclusions so entirely opposite to those of a large majority of independent observers.

During the Doctor's residence in Hankow we find he treated no fewer than 993 cases for opium smoking; all, except 25, were in-door patients. In the reports for 1876-7 we find that " broken health " is one of the main reasons which the patients gave for wishing to relinquish the habit; while in the report for 1878 Dr. Mackenzie, writing of the difficulty in giving up the habit, sums up his experience of 993 cases in these words : " The habit of opium smoking, prolonged for any length of time, plays

havoc with the man's natural energy, rendering him indolent and enervated. Few in this condition can, unaided,
combat the craving for opium and effectually reform.
The attempt is often made, but as often ends in disappointment. For a time they persevere, but when the intolerable
craving, accompanied by extreme bodily depression, with
violent achings of the joints and muscular pains, sets in,
they fly to their old enemy, and drown themselves in
opium stupor." The reference to this subject concludes
with a typical illustration of the kind of case generally
seeking admission into opium refuges. " A man of twenty-
five, emaciated and feeble, . . . a fortune-teller, with once
a thriving business, who took to opium smoking, which led
to disastrous results. His earnings were squandered and
his health was broken down." The line of treatment
adopted is concisely put in the report for 1878 : " There
is no medicinal specific guaranteed to cure ; the object
aimed at is to relieve symptoms as they arise, and so to
help the patient back to health and freedom."

Passing on to review the pre-eminently successful labours
of Mackenzie in Tien-tsin, we note, in the first place, a
general similarity in the nature of medical and surgical
cases met with in Hankow and Tien-tsin. We have not,
however, sufficient data for drawing any reliable conclusions as to the comparative frequency of the various diseases
treated in the two districts, and must accordingly content
ourselves with calling attention—

(1) To the out-door patients' statistics.
(2) To the in-door patients' statistics.
(3) To the statistics of operations performed.

(1) *Out-door Patients' Statistics.*

During the first five and a half months' work in the city,
under the support of the Viceroy, Li Hung Chang, 3,174
new cases were seen, 10,552 visits paid by them, and, in

addition, 3,405 opium smokers received treatment as out-door patients.

The report of this work yields the following interesting facts :—

Diseases of Respiratory System	318	cases.
„ Alimentary System	314	„
„ Cutaneous System	248	„
„ Eye Diseases	216	„
„ Nervous System, etc., etc. . .	146	„

While of individual diseases we have the following figures :—

Dyspepsia	157	cases.
Chronic Rheumatism	129	„
Asthma	106	„
Tinea Tonsurans	101	„
Bronchitis	91	„
Ulcers	86	„
Syphilis	68	„
Eczema	65	„
Dysentery	59	„
Sciatica	58	„
Intermittent Fever, etc., etc.	45	„

The results of Dr. Mackenzie's extensive efforts in Tien-tsin to treat opium-smokers successfully as out-door patients, by means of gradually diminishing doses of opium or its alkaloid, morphia, are highly instructive, especially since they were arrived at after ten and a half months' treatment of such cases, during which time he prescribed for no fewer than 5,106.

We find he gave up the practice, being convinced that such a line of treatment was, in the vast majority of cases, powerless to effect a cure. By a cure we mean not only that the patient no longer smokes opium, but also that he no longer requires to take the opium-containing remedy.

(2) *In-door Patients' Statistics.*

This department of the work the Doctor long felt to be

the most valuable and satisfactory. The average attendance of an out-patient was two to four days, which in many cases meant that the patient was unable or unwilling to give foreign medicine a more lengthy trial. On the other hand, the average stay of an in-door patient was about three weeks, implying more satisfactory treatment and better results in most cases, while in addition it gave the patient an opportunity of learning many of the vital truths of the Gospel and the possibility of spiritual as well as physical healing.

The nature and extent of Dr. Mackenzie's work among his in-door patients may be gathered from the following statement of cases treated in one year. An examination of it reveals many interesting facts, *e.g.*, the great preponderance of " eye cases," especially of entropion, leucoma, and granular conjunctivitis ; also of necrosis, fistula in ano, and dyspepsia. We also notice the large number of cures or improvements obtained, and the small number of deaths.

STATEMENT OF CASES TREATED IN THE WARDS OF THE VICEROY'S HOSPITAL, TIEN-TSIN, FROM JANUARY IST TO DECEMBER 31ST, 1886.

Diseases.	Number Admitted.	Cured or Relieved.	Unrelieved.	Died.
General Diseases. **28** *cases.*				
Remittent Fever . .	7	7		
Intermittent Fever . .	2	2		
Tertiary Syphilis . .	5	5		
Rheumatism, Subacute .	5	5		
,, Chronic . .	8	8		
Measles	1	1		
Diseases of the Nervous System. **34** *cases.*				
Epilepsy	6	6		
Spinal Neuralgia . . .	2	2		
Hemiplegia	3	1	2	
Paraplegia	1	1		
Paralysis (local) . . .	8	8		

Disease.	Number Admitted.	Cured or Relieved.	Unrelieved.	Died.
Chorea	2	I	I	
Tic Douloureux . . .	I		I	
Locomotor Ataxy . . .	I	I		
Sciatica	10	10		
Diseases of the Circulatory System. **9** *cases.*				
Valvular Disease of Heart .	5	4		I
Subclavian Aneurism . .	1		I	
Varicose Veins . . .	I	I		
Arteritis (causing gangrene of foot)	2	2		
Diseases of the Respiratory System. **38** *cases.*				
Bronchitis	17	17		
Pneumonia	4	4		
Phthisis	10	10		
Pleurisy	4	4		
Asthma, Spasmodic . .	I	I		
Laryngitis	I	I		
Empyema	I			I
Diseases of the Digestive System. **78** *cases.*				
Dyspepsia	27	27		
Dysentery	9	7	2	
Abscess of Liver . . .	I	I		
Cancer of Stomach . .	I	I		
Gall Stone Colic . . .	2	2		
Hepatitis	I	I		
Peritonitis	I	I		
Fistula in Ano . . .	26	26		
Ascites	2	2		
Hæmorrhoids . . .	8	8		
Diseases of the Genito-Urinary Organs. **26** *cases.*				
Spermatorrhœa . . .	2	2		
Phymosis	7	7		
Urethral Stricture . .	7	6		I
Orchitis	I	I		
Nephritis	4	3		I
Varicocele	I	I		
Incontinence of Urine . .	I	I		
Cystitis	2	2		
Calculus in Bladder . .	I	I		

Disease.	Number Admitted.	Cured or Relieved.	Unrelieved.	Died.
Diseases of the Bones and Joints. **41** *cases.*				
Necrosis	28	28		
Synovitis of Knee and Shoulder	6	6		
Hip-joint Disease. . .	2	2		
Arthritis of Knee . . .	2	1		1
,, ,, Elbow . .	1	1		
Sprained Ankle . . .	1	1		
Anchylosis	1	1		
Diseases of the Skin. **34** *cases.*				
Eczema	3	3		
Psoriasis	8	8		
Carbuncle	1	1		
Rodent Ulcer and Lupus .	3	2		
Ulcers	15	15		
Burns by Kerosene . .	1			1
Gangrene (from frost bite) .	3	3	1	
Diseases of the Eye. **164** *cases.*				
Ectropion	2	2		
Entropion and Trichiasis .	57	57		
Pterygium	11	11		
Glaucoma	13	12		
Leucoma	21	21	1	
Closed Pupil after Iritis .	8	5		
Cataract	12	11	3	
Conjunctivitis Catarrhal .	2	2	1	
,, Granular .	21	21		
,, Purulent .	2	2		
,, Pustular .	1	1		
Corneitis	5	5		
Ulcers of Cornea . . .	5	5		
Hypopion	1	1		
Ophthalmia Tarsi . .	1	1		
Retinitis	2		1	
Injuries. **29** *cases.*				
Fractures (1 compound of thigh, 1 old ununited) .	4	2	2	
Dislocations	4	4		
Gun-Shot Wounds . .	6	5		
Contused and Lacerated Wounds	14	14		1
Cut Throat	1	1		

Disease.	Number Admitted.	Cured or Relieved.	Unrelieved.	Died.
Miscellaneous. **76** *cases.*				
Tumours, Simple . . .	12	12		
,, Malignant . .	12	12		
Nasal Polypi . . .	2	2		
Abscesses (Perinephritic 2)	16	16		
Sinuses and Fistulæ . .	21	21		
Hare-lip	8	8		
Unclassified	5	5		

Summary of In-patients.

General Diseases	28	cases
Nervous System	34	,,
Circulatory System	9	,,
Respiratory System	38	,,
Digestive System	78	,,
Genito-Urinary System	26	,,
Bones and Joints	41	,,
Skin	33	,,
Eye	164	,,
Injuries	29	,,
Miscellaneous	76	,,
Total . . .	556	

556 in-patients, each averaging 21½ days' residence in hospital. Average number of patients in the wards during the year, 42. Seven deaths.

(3) *Statistics of Operations Performed.*

Nothing could be more suggestive as to the growth of the Tien-tsin medical mission work than a comparison of the number of operations performed during the first and last years of Dr. Mackenzie's career. During the first year, when he had no in-door accommodation and only a very limited staff of native assistants, the operations, though by no means few, were all of a minor nature, the larger number being for hare-lip, 23 ; for tumours, 20 ; for pterygium, 14 ; and for entropion, 32. In striking contrast to this is the tabulated list given below of opera-

tions performed in 1886, some of which will be seen to
have been of the most serious nature.

These statistics speak loudly of Dr. Mackenzie s well-
earned reputation, and of the implicit confidence placed in
him by those who submitted themselves for treatment;
while they also indicate the high state of development the
work had attained to through the blessing of God, which
so manifestly rested on the indefatigable labours of His
servant.

VICEROY'S HOSPITAL, TIEN-TSIN. LIST OF SURGICAL OPERATIONS
PERFORMED FROM JANUARY 1ST TO DECEMBER 31ST, 1886.

Total 589.

Eye Operations. **212** *cases.*   Cases

Ptcrygium (excised or transplanted)	35
Ectropion	2
Entropion	94
Iridectomy for Artificial Pupil	43
„ „ Glaucoma	16
Cataract	17
Strabismus	2
Paracentesis Cornea.	3

Amputations. **24** *cases.*

„ of Forcarm	3
„ „ Thumb	2
„ „ Fingers	5
„ „ Leg	1
„ „ Foot { Pirogoff's . . 3 / Syme's . . 1 / Chopart's . . 1 }	5
„ „ Toes	3
„ „ Penis (for Epithelioma) . . .	5
Excisions of Knee Joint	2
„ „ Portion of Rib	1
„ „ Metatarsal Bone of Foot . . .	2
Removal of Tumours	37
„ „ Toe Nails	2
„ „ Uvula	
„ „ Nasal Polypi	2
Extraction of Bullet from Thigh	2
Lithotomy (supra pubic operation)	1

Fistula in Ano 32
Hare-lip 8
Hæmorrhoids, External 5

                (Ligatured . 4)
   „   Internal { Clamp . . 1 } . . . 6
                (Nitric Acid . 1)

Fissure of Anus 1
Circumcision for Phymosis 7
Hydrocele tapped 5
Varicocele (radical cure) 1
Varicose Veins (radical cure) 1
Operations for Necrosed Bone 31
Puncture of Bladder (supra pubic, for retention with
   bad stricture) 5
External Urethrotomy 3
Nævus destroyed with Thermo-Cautery 1
Wiring Ununited Fracture 1
Scraping Lupus and Rodent Ulcers 5
Extraction of Needles and Splinters 3
Operation for Paraphymosis 1
Splitting up Sinuses 27
Breaking down Adhesions in Joints 4
Abscesses opened (many antiseptically opened and
   drained, 2 Perinephritic) 77
Abscess of Liver (antiseptically opened and drained) . 1
Operation for Carbuncle 16
Paracentesis Thoracis 16
   „   Abdominis 30

Dislocation reduced. **8 cases.**

        Hip 2
        Shoulder 3
        Elbow 2
        Thumb 1

Fractures treated. **8 cases.**

        Clavicle 1
        Humerus 1
        Ulna 1
        Femur 3
        Tibia and Fibula 1
        Fibula 1

                Total . . 589

III.

THE EVANGELISTIC SIDE OF A MEDICAL MISSION.

BY J. KENNETH MACKENZIE, M.R.C.S., L.R.C.P.

THE medical missionary comes to China to advance the cause of Christ. This is fully admitted. But there is not the same unanimity of opinion as to *how* he can best advance his Saviour's cause. Many contend that his province is to confine himself to the healing of the sick, the training of medical students, and in the course of years, perhaps, adding to his multifarious duties the translation or preparation of medical works ; meanwhile, showing general sympathy in Christian effort, but leaving to his clerical colleagues the work of evangelization. Others, again, think that he should personally take part in, if not superintend, the spiritual work amongst his patients—in fact, be at the head of the evangelists as well as the medical department of the Medical Mission. Such a view does not imply that he is not ready to welcome all the help he can get from his clerical brethren. The following remarks are written to advocate this latter opinion. There are two main objections generally brought forward against it. The first, that a jack-of-all-trades is a master of none, and that consequently you cannot have a good doctor and a good parson in the same individual. This is quite true. But I am not advocating the making of parsons ; indeed I would wish to see every medical missionary come out unordained, and it is not necessary that he should ever directly engage in preaching. To answer the other objection, viz., that he hasn't time, I would reply, that the old saying, " Where there's a will there's a way," holds good here. He must *make time*, for his business is only half done if he neglects this portion of it. How then can the evangelistic side of a Medical Mission best be developed ?

The prevailing opinion seems to be in favour of establishing in connection with every such mission, as soon as possible, a hospital with ward accommodation for in-patients. It is evident upon the surface that the best medical work can be achieved in this way, and there cannot be two opinions, where the experiment has been fairly tried, that the walls of an hospital give about the best opportunity to be found anywhere for direct personal dealing with men's souls. A statement one commonly hears made by clerical missionaries is to the effect, that in chapel preaching to the heathen the difficulty is to get in touch with the people, to approach them as individuals. The preacher deals with his audience in the mass. We, in our hospital, on the other hand, can come into direct personal contact with men. Our relationship as doctor and patient removes at once the sense of separation, amounting oftentimes to actual hostility, shown by individual Chinese when approached by the foreigner.

One of the best ways in which the medical missionary can influence his patients is by keeping up the spiritual life of his assistants, encouraging them to prayer and the frequent study of the Scriptures. Of course, he can only aid them as he is himself abiding in Christ, and drawing strength and life from his Saviour. He cannot give what he has not himself got. The knowledge of this should stimulate us to a constant and close walk with God. It is of little account for us to pray for the outpouring of the Holy Spirit upon our assistants or patients, until the great cry of our hearts is, " Lord, fill me ! " and then, when we are full, from us will go forth streams of living water to those around. Experience has taught me not to employ any men *specially* for religious work. The helpers should all be converted men, and *they* should carry the gospel to the patients under the supervision of the doctor. By helpers I mean dispensers who assist in the compounding of drugs, and ward attendants or dressers, who correspond, in the work they do, to our nurses at home.

I can best set forth my ideas on the subject by describing our own practice. During the year 1886 there was an average of 42 in-patients daily in our wards, with an average length of residence for each of 21½ days. These patients pay for their own food and provide bedding, excepting in a few instances, such as severe accident cases. We employ two dispensers, three ward attendants, a cook, gatekeeper, coolie,—all but the last being working Christians.

We begin the day with a Bible reading, at which the helpers and most of the convalescent patients are present. It usually lasts about three-quarters of an hour, and is made as conversational as possible by asking and soliciting questions, and inducing as many as are willing to take part. People enjoy a meeting much more when they have some part in it, however small. Above all things, the leader should avoid " preaching " if the meeting is to be interesting and profitable.

Most of our medical work in the wards is done before two o'clock, so that the ward attendants are able to spend a large portion of every day in teaching the catechism to those patients who are both well enough and willing to receive instruction. With a little management and encouragement from the doctor an enthusiasm can be aroused, and the more advanced among the patients will help in instructing the others. " How shall they believe in Him of whom they have not heard ? " On Tuesday evenings we hold a class, in which we try to gather up the work of the week, "drawing up the gospel net," as it has well been termed ; and on Friday evenings there is a special meeting for the helpers and other Christians for prayer and the study of the Scriptures, the medical missionary being the leader at these various classes.

I want to set forth a few reasons *why* the medical man should himself engage in evangelistic work.

First.—He can best influence his own patients.

They are looking to him for relief from suffering, and if he is doing his best to succour them, and they see that he is equally interested in their spiritual state, they will, out of sheer desire to please, begin to pay attention to these matters. This may seem a low motive, but never mind what is the motive if only the interest. Many a man is aroused has gone to a revival meeting to scoff and has remained to pray.

Second.—His assistants will be, under God, largely what he makes them.

It is a common statement at home that a Church is what its pastor is. Has he the missionary spirit? Then the Church will be a Missionary Church. Is he an aggressive man? Then the Church will be a Working Church. It is a trite saying, and yet one we often seem to forget, that men are taught by practice rather than by precept. It is of little use for the doctor to urge his assistants to Christian work while he himself is showing but lukewarm interest, or none at all. He must teach " do as I do " rather than "do as I say."

Third.—Unless he attends to it, the full value of the Medical Mission as a Christianizing Agency will not be developed.

It is no disparagement to our clerical colleagues to say this, for their main energies must necessarily be devoted to church organization and public teaching.

Fourth.—His own spiritual life requires it.

If the life of the soul is to be anything more than a name; if it is to remain in a healthy condition, it must needs find a channel for its activity. " We cannot but speak the things which we have seen and heard."

Then, too, there are so many depressing influences surrounding him in his medical work. The daily drudgery of the out-patient clinic, with its crowd of sick folk, becomes at times trying to the flesh. A medical visitor once said to me, " How *can* you spend your life amongst these dirty wretches ? " And in the wards, though to the lover of his profession there is much to attract in the study of cases of special interest, yet there is also much to weary. He has to work with imperfect instruments in the shape of clumsy if willing men, in place of the intelligent and tender nurses of our home hospitals. He has to put up with ideas of cleanliness that do not always accord with his own. All these things tend to depress a man. We need the elevating influence of service for God to counterbalance this state. When we aim at winning the souls of our patients to Christ, we begin to find how dreadfully dead to spiritual things the Chinese are, and how true it is that we can do nothing without the Holy Spirit, whose it is to convince of sin ; and this knowledge drives us to prayer, that He, who is the Quickener of the dead, may come into *our* lives and work, and then we shall have the joy of seeing the light break in upon the souls of our patients, and we ourselves will be raised above the drudgery of our daily toil, and our work will become ennobling to our higher nature.

Tien-tsin *March 4th,* 1887.

IV.

THE DOUBLE CURE.

THE medical missionary has this great advantage over his clerical brother, that the people seek him, he has not to trouble about seeking them ; and yet they come only for the material benefits he can confer upon them in the healing of the diseases of the body.

It was the same in our Lord's day ; the great majority of those who sought to see Jesus came only for bodily healing ; very few indeed sought Him, in the first place, for spiritual aid. And so we find Him, while daily surrounded by a multitude of people, exclaiming, " Ye will not come to Me that ye might have life." Our Lord was one day on the way to the house of Jairus, with a thronging crowd surging about Him, when into the midst crept a frail woman, who had suffered for twelve years from a painful disorder. Timidly she pushed her way through the crowd to get near Jesus, and then stretching forth her hand she touched His garment. There was much pushing and squeezing around Him, but He felt only one touch, and that was the hand of the poor helpless woman in her extremity. This touch of faith delighted and cheered the Saviour's heart.

Let us not be satisfied with mere crowds flocking to us for medical treatment. We have a higher vocation to fulfil. Let us wait expectingly for this *touch of faith,* and with the Master may this alone satisfy our hearts.

Our waiting-room may be full of patients, and all our beds be occupied, and yet these men and women will pass from under our care, pretty much as they came to us, so far as higher things are concerned, unless we directly bestir ourselves for their spiritual good. They seek us, it is true, but for their bodies only ; if we would win their souls, we must *seek them.* The command to us, as to all disciples, is " Go ye "—" Compel them to come in." Deliver us from thinking that we are obeying this command when we employ an evangelist and say to him, " *You* go and preach to the patients, while *I* attend to their bodies." *This* is not being a medical missionary.

Let us look at our great ideal medical missionary—the Lord Jesus Christ. What were His methods ? When Nicodemus, the man of position, of unblemished moral

26

character in the eyes of the world, sought the Lord for some friendly conversation one evening, Jesus takes up the theme, "Ye must be born again." When the respectable man, the official perhaps, visits us to return thanks for medical help, or to see some of the wonders from Western lands which we may have to show him, the Lord help us to be faithful to our commission. We may by so doing offend him,—and no doubt Nicodemus was offended at first by the direct personal dealing of our Lord. Yet what of that? it is ours to obey, it is His to provide. We have in mind a rich patient, an official, who, when spoken to concerning Jesus, uttered some very bitter things against our Saviour's name, and was even inclined to argue against Christianity, but who later on sent five hundred taels for our hospital; and when, a year after, he called, bringing with him a friend to see the wards, he challenged his friend that if he, the friend, would give five hundred taels, he himself would repeat his former donation. The challenge was accepted, and a thousand taels was added to our fund that day. Again he brought another friend to see the hospital, and persuaded him to give a donation of three hundred taels. Having been under treatment some two or three years later, he sent a third donation of five hundred taels. Thus the Lord, through the agency of this former opponent of Christianity, provided us with two thousand three hundred taels. Depend upon it, we never injure our cause by our faithfulness; it is just the other way.

So, too, when they brought to Him the palsied man lying on his bed, it is of his spiritual state Jesus thinks first, and thus He says, " Thy sins are forgiven thee."

Should we not seek to imitate the Lord's method, even though the result be but a very feeble copy of the great original? What is it that we have to impart? Let us be definite with ourselves. Is it some new dogma? a system of doctrine from the West? If so, by all means leave the religious element in the hands of the evangelist;

he will expound your doctrines better than you can. But we reject such an idea. The Chinese have already more than enough of mere empty doctrine. What we bring them is no lifeless form, but a living personal Saviour whom it is our privilege to present to the Chinese; and this glorious privilege of representing our Saviour King, and witnessing for HIM, we *dare not* commit to any second party.

When we go our rounds in the wards we examine into the cases before us, and prescribe the remedies according to the best of our ability. We omit nothing within our reach which can help our patients. We are lavish with costly restoratives if they are necessary to the saving of the man's life. But herein are we different from hundreds of medical men in other parts of the world who owe no allegiance to Jesus, and yet who spare neither strength, time, nor money in the enthusiasm of hospital work. The difference should lie in the fact that we are *as* thorough, *as* definite in seeking the cure of the soul's malady, as they and we alike are in succouring the bodies of men.

Our remedies frequently fail, but Christ, as the remedy for sin, never fails. It is true it often *seems* to fail, but the reason is that the remedy is not properly applied. It is our great lamentation that the Chinese are so negligent in regularly following up treatment. A man takes one or two doses of medicine, and because he is not distinctly better as a consequence, he declares the foreign doctor cannot cure him, and ceases to attend. Have our medicines failed in this case? Certainly not. And so, though sometimes discouraged, we yet persevere, having faith that we can accomplish good, and that our work must tell in time. Now let us act in the same way with this spiritual malady *sin.*

The first essential is that the patient recognises the fact that he is sick, else he certainly will not take the medicine. We must press home this truth with all our might. Then, too, we need to pray more for and with our patients, and to labour on with thankful and restful hearts, knowing that as surely as the rain comes down from heaven to moisten and fertilize the earth, so certainly will the Holy Spirit be poured out upon our patients, causing the Word to take root in their hearts and to bring forth fruit in their lives.

But some will say, It is impossible to find time for this double work. We beg leave to differ from them. The medical missionary who is at the head of a large hospital should be like a master-workman, overseeing everything, setting each his task, while reserving to himself the delicate and important workmanship. We would have him do less work perhaps, but work of a higher quality. Do not let him spend his strength in seeing vast crowds of out-patients, when the statistics of many hospitals combine to show that scarcely more than two visits are paid by each individual, and therefore from a medical standpoint alone the results are most unsatisfactory. This department must be kept up, but let him leave it largely in the hands of trained assistants, he himself doing well that which is best worth the doing.